Katja Franke

BrainAGE

Katja Franke

BrainAGE

A novel machine learning approach for identifying abnormal age-related brain changes

Südwestdeutscher Verlag für Hochschulschriften

Impressum / Imprint
Bibliografische Information der Deutschen Nationalbibliothek: Die Deutsche Nationalbibliothek verzeichnet diese Publikation in der Deutschen Nationalbibliografie; detaillierte bibliografische Daten sind im Internet über http://dnb.d-nb.de abrufbar.
Alle in diesem Buch genannten Marken und Produktnamen unterliegen warenzeichen-, marken- oder patentrechtlichem Schutz bzw. sind Warenzeichen oder eingetragene Warenzeichen der jeweiligen Inhaber. Die Wiedergabe von Marken, Produktnamen, Gebrauchsnamen, Handelsnamen, Warenbezeichnungen u.s.w. in diesem Werk berechtigt auch ohne besondere Kennzeichnung nicht zu der Annahme, dass solche Namen im Sinne der Warenzeichen- und Markenschutzgesetzgebung als frei zu betrachten wären und daher von jedermann benutzt werden dürften.

Bibliographic information published by the Deutsche Nationalbibliothek: The Deutsche Nationalbibliothek lists this publication in the Deutsche Nationalbibliografie; detailed bibliographic data are available in the Internet at http://dnb.d-nb.de.
Any brand names and product names mentioned in this book are subject to trademark, brand or patent protection and are trademarks or registered trademarks of their respective holders. The use of brand names, product names, common names, trade names, product descriptions etc. even without a particular marking in this works is in no way to be construed to mean that such names may be regarded as unrestricted in respect of trademark and brand protection legislation and could thus be used by anyone.

Coverbild / Cover image: www.ingimage.com

Verlag / Publisher:
Südwestdeutscher Verlag für Hochschulschriften
ist ein Imprint der / is a trademark of
OmniScriptum GmbH & Co. KG
Heinrich-Böcking-Str. 6-8, 66121 Saarbrücken, Deutschland / Germany
Email: info@svh-verlag.de

Herstellung: siehe letzte Seite /
Printed at: see last page
ISBN: 978-3-8381-3346-1

Zugl. / Approved by: Zürich, UZH, Diss., 2013

Copyright © 2014 OmniScriptum GmbH & Co. KG
Alle Rechte vorbehalten. / All rights reserved. Saarbrücken 2014

Danksagung

Zuallererst möchte ich meinem Doktorvater Dr. Christian Gaser für die exzellente und kompetente, aber nichtsdestoweniger herzliche und humorvolle Betreuung danken. Christian, ich danke Dir insbesondere für die vielen geistreichen Gespräche, Deine unermüdliche Geduld und Dein Vertrauen in mich! Ich möchte mich herzlich bei Prof. Lutz Jäncke bedanken, der es mir ermöglicht hat, an der Universität Zürich zu promovieren – trotz einiger organisatorischer Hürden. Weiterhin möchte ich mich bei meinen Kollegen der *Structural Brain Mapping Group* bedanken: Rachel Yotter, ich danke Dir für deinen unermüdlichen Einsatz, mein Englisch zu polieren, und für verrückte Freitagnachmittage. Robert Dahnke, ich danke dir für deine perfekte Organisation all der kleinen und großen Dinge, deine Erste Hilfe in all den nervigen Computerdingen und dafür, dass du immer ein nettes Wort auf den Lippen hast. Gabriel Ziegler, ich danke Dir für all die interessanten und herausfordernden Diskussionen. Alissa Winkler, ich danke Dir für Deine vielen hilfreichen Kommentare. Insbesondere möchte ich Gerrit Röbisch, meiner Familie und all denjenigen danken, die mich immer wieder liebevoll unterstützt, mich hin und wieder abgelenkt und unerschütterlich an mich geglaubt haben.
Emil, Anton, Paul – Danke, dass es Euch gibt!

Contents

Abstract	**5**
Zusammenfassung	**7**
1 General Introduction	**9**
1.1 Age-related changes of the human brain structure	9
1.2 Variability in brain aging	11
1.3 Associations of brain structures with cognitive functions	13
1.4 Accelerated brain atrophy in neurodegenerative diseases	15
1.5 The *BrainAGE* approach	20
2 Estimating the age of healthy subjects from T1-weighted MRI scans using kernel methods: Exploring the influence of various parameters	**23**
2.1 Abstract	23
2.2 Introduction	24
2.3 Methods	28
2.3.1 Subjects / database	28
2.3.2 Preprocessing of structural MRI data	29
2.3.3 Data reduction	30
2.3.4 Support vector regression (SVR)	31
2.3.5 Relevance vector regression (RVR)	32
2.3.6 Computing the age estimation model	33
2.3.7 Systematic analyses of different parameters influencing the age estimation model	34
2.3.8 Application of the age estimation framework to data from the ADNI database	37
2.4 Results	38
2.4.1 Performance measures	38
2.4.2 Influence of different scanners	39
2.4.3 Impact of regression methods and data reduction	40

	2.4.4 Comparison of variations in data preprocessing (affine vs. modulated, smoothing, and spatial resolution)	43
	2.4.5 Influence of the size of training data	44
	2.4.6 Comparing the influence of the various parameters	45
	2.4.7 Estimating the age of patients with early AD	46
2.5	Discussion	46

3 Longitudinal changes in individual *BrainAGE* in healthy aging, mild cognitive impairment, and Alzheimer's disease   **53**

3.1	Abstract	53
3.2	Introduction	53
3.3	Methods	56
	3.3.1 ADNI database	56
	3.3.2 Subjects	57
	3.3.3 Preprocessing of MRI data and data reduction	59
	3.3.4 *BrainAGE* framework	59
	3.3.5 Statistical analysis	60
3.4	Results	61
	3.4.1 Stability of *BrainAGE* estimations	61
	3.4.2 Longitudinal *BrainAGE* estimation	63
3.5	Discussion	67

4 Advanced *BrainAGE* in older adults with type 2 diabetes mellitus   **72**

4.1	Abstract	72
4.2	Introduction	73
4.3	Research design and methods	75
	4.3.1 Subjects	75
	4.3.2 Magnetic resonance imaging (MRI)	78
	4.3.3 Preprocessing of MRI data and data reduction	78
	4.3.4 Age estimation framework	79
	4.3.5 Statistical analysis	80

4.4	Results	82
	4.4.1 Group characteristics	82
	4.4.2 Cross-sectional *BrainAGE* analyses	82
	4.4.3 Longitudinal *BrainAGE* analyses	85
4.5	Discussion	86
5	***BrainAGE* in mild cognitive impaired patients: Predicting the conversion to Alzheimer's disease**	**93**
5.1	Abstract	93
5.2	Background	94
5.3	Methods	96
	5.3.1 Subjects	96
	5.3.2 Preprocessing of MRI data and data reduction	98
	5.3.3 Relevance vector regression (RVR)	100
	5.3.4 Age estimation framework	101
	5.3.5 Statistical analysis	102
5.4	Results	104
	5.4.1 Whole MCI sample	104
	5.4.2 MCI subsample with CSF data	109
5.5	Discussion	110
6	**General Discussion**	**124**
6.1	Stability of *BrainAGE* estimation	124
	6.1.1 Limitations of the *BrainAGE* approach	127
6.2	Application of the *BrainAGE* approach to clinical samples	128
	6.2.1 Associations of *BrainAGE* with cognitive functions	131
	6.2.2 Prediction of prospective conversion to AD using *BrainAGE*	132
7	**Conclusions and perspectives**	**135**
References		**137**

Abstract

Early identification of neuroanatomical changes deviating from the normal age-related atrophy pattern has the potential to improve clinical outcomes through early treatment or prophylaxis. Especially the pathological cascade of Alzheimer's disease (AD), the most common form of dementia, is widely linked to precocious and / or accelerated (brain) aging.

This work presents a novel magnetic resonance imaging (MRI)-based biomarker that indicates discrepancies in individual brain aging and even predicts prospective cognitive decline. By employing automatic preprocessing of structural MR images as well as high-dimensional pattern recognition methods, the *BrainAGE* approach uses the distribution of normal brain-aging patterns to estimate the brain age of a given new subject. The difference between the estimated and the chronological age is termed the *"Brain Age Gap Estimation"* (*BrainAGE*) score, with positive values indicating the degree of acceleration in cerebral atrophy, which is considered a risk factor for AD.

The *BrainAGE* approach proved to be a reliable, scanner-independent, and efficient method for brain age estimation in healthy subjects, yielding a correlation of $r = 0.92$ between the chronological and the estimated brain age. Moreover, with significantly increased *BrainAGE* scores in AD patients, in subjects who converted to AD during follow-up, and even in subjects with diabetes mellitus type 2 (T2DM), the *BrainAGE* framework demonstrated its potential to indicate accelerated brain aging. Additionally, increased *BrainAGE* scores were profoundly associated with disease severity and prospective worsening of cognitive functions.

Most clinically valuable, the *BrainAGE* outperformed all cognitive scales, hippocampus volume, and state-of-the-art biomarkers derived from cerebrospinal fluid (CSF) in predicting prospective conversion to AD. Furthermore, each additional year in the *BrainAGE* score was associated with a nearly 10% greater risk of developing AD within the next 36 months.

In conclusion, the *BrainAGE* approach showed promising results on an individual level, contributing to an early detection of abnormal brain aging, and providing important prognostic information. Its fast and fully automated nature facilitates the integration into the clinical workflow, thus qualifying as a tool for screening as well as for monitoring treatment options.

Zusammenfassung

Die frühzeitige Identifikation neuro-anatomischer Veränderungen, die vom normalen Atrophiemuster abweichen, kann klinische Prognosen durch eine frühzeitige Behandlung oder Prophylaxe verbessern. Insbesondere die Alzheimer Demenz (AD), die häufigste Art der Demenz, scheint mit einer vorzeitigen und / oder beschleunigten (Gehirn-) Alterung zusammen zu hängen. Diese Arbeit präsentiert einen neuartigen Magnetresonanztomographie (MRI)-gestützten Biomarker, der auf Abweichungen in der individuellen Gehirnalterung hinweist und kognitiven Verfall voraussagt. Mittels automatisierter Vorverarbeitung von strukturellen MRI-Daten sowie hochdimensionaler Mustererkennungsmethoden modelliert der *BrainAGE*-Ansatz den Verlauf von normaler Gehirnalterung. Anschließend kann das Gehirnalter eines neuen Probanden geschätzt werden. Die Differenz zwischen dem geschätzten und dem chronologischen Alter wird *"Brain Age Gap Estimation"* (*BrainAGE*) genannt, wobei positive Werte den Grad der Beschleunigung in der Gehirnatrophie anzeigen und somit auf ein erhöhtes Risiko für AD hinweisen.

Mit einer Korrelation von $r = 0.92$ zwischen dem chronologischen und dem geschätzten Gehirnalter in einer Gruppe gesunder Probanden hat sich der *BrainAGE*-Ansatz als eine zuverlässige, Scanner-unabhängige und effiziente Methode für die Schätzung des Gehirnalters erwiesen. Mit signifikant erhöhten *BrainAGE*-Werten in AD-Patienten, in Probanden, die während des follow-ups zu AD konvertieren, und sogar in Patienten mit Diabetes mellitus Typ 2 (T2DM), hat die *BrainAGE*-Methode außerdem sein Potenzial demonstriert, beschleunigte Gehirnalterung zu identifizieren. Weiterhin gehen erhöhte *BrainAGE*-Werte mit dem Schweregrad der AD-Symptome und mit der zukünftigen Verschlechterung kognitiver Funktionen einher.

Im Vergleich zu verschiedenen kognitiven Tests, zum Hippocampus-Volumen und zu den state-of-the-art Biomarkern aus der cerebrospinalen

Flüssigkeit (CSF) hat die *BrainAGE*-Methode eine zukünftiger Konvertierung zu AD am genauesten vorhergesagt. Jedes zusätzliche Jahr in den *BrainAGE*-Werten war mit einem ca. 10% grösseren Risiko verbunden, innerhalb der nächsten 36 Monate zu AD zu konvertieren.

Somit stellt die *BrainAGE*-Methode einen vielversprechende Ansatz dar, abweichende Muster in der individuellen Gehirnalterung frühzeitig festzustellen und wichtige prognostische Informationen zu liefern. Da die *BrainAGE*-Methode schnell und völlig automatisiert arbeitet, könnte sie zukünftig beispielsweise als Screeninginstrument oder zur Bewertung von Behandlungserfolgen in den klinischen Arbeitsablauf integriert werden.

Chapter 1.
General Introduction

"If the brain were so simple we could understand it, we would be so simple we couldn't."
(Lyall Watson)

Understanding the brain, and in particular understanding the processes occurring during healthy as well as abnormal brain aging, is one of the intriguing questions of mankind. This chapter outlines the general context in which the *BrainAGE* approach was developed and implemented. First, neuroanatomical insights into normal brain aging are briefly reviewed. Then, diverse variables are described that influence neurodegenerative processes and therefore add to the variability seen in age-related brain changes. Some of these variables are supposed to lead to accelerated brain atrophy that shows the pattern of faster brain aging. Finally, research findings are summarized suggesting that processes of accelerated brain aging will make the brain more vulnerable to neurodegenerative diseases, especially Alzheimer's disease (AD).

1.1 Age-related changes of the human brain structure

Postmortem and histological studies of the human brain have discovered a wide range of age-related changes in brain structure (Raz and Rodrigue, 2006). Amongst others, reduced brain weight and volume as well as sulcal expansion were revealed on a coarse level (Kemper, 1994; Pakkenberg and Gundersen, 1997; Skullerud, 1985). Research at cellular levels also detected several atrophy processes, including loss of neocortical neurons over the life span by about 10% in both sexes (Pakkenberg and Gundersen, 1997), decrease in the number of neurons in the hippocampal formation (Simic et al., 1997) and the cerebellum (Ellis, 1920), decline of the white matter (WM) structure, with a primary loss of thinner fibers and a relative preservation of the thicker ones (Marner et al., 2003; Meier-Ruge et al., 1992), reduction in synaptic density (Morrison and Hof, 1997), deafferentation within the hippocampus (Bertoni-Freddari et al., 2002), and significant loss of dendritic spines (Jacobs et al., 1997). Taken together, although some age-related changes are affecting the brain globally, most findings suggest a rather region- and layer-specific reduction (Uylings and de Brabander, 2002).

But it was only after the advent of magnetic resonance imaging (MRI) that neuroimaging studies contributed to a better understanding of brain aging – especially when it comes to longitudinal studies, which were obviously not possible to conduct before. In addition, with the availability of automated computational methods for analyzing MRI data, such as voxel-based morphometry (VBM; Ashburner and Friston, 2000), it has become feasible to quantify and visualize structural brain changes in vivo (May, 2011).

Healthy brain aging has been found to follow highly coordinated and sequenced patterns. Pfefferbaum et al. (1994) showed that gray matter (GM) volume increases from birth until the age of four and thereafter decreases continuously until subjects reach their 70's, while WM volume increases steadily until around the age of 20 when it plateaus. Cerebrospinal fluid (CSF) was found to exhibit a complementary pattern, remaining constant until about 20 years of age and increasing steadily thereafter (Pfefferbaum et al., 1994).

The pattern of linear GM decline and CSF increase being predominant in normal aging is also supported by a more recent, fully automated VBM study (Good et al., 2001). Furthermore, local areas of accelerated GM decline and microstructural changes in WM were reported, suggesting a heterogeneous and complex pattern of atrophy across the adult life span (Good et al., 2001). Evidence for more region-specific and non-linear patterns of neurodegenerative age-related changes in GM volume were provided by cross-sectional morphometric analyses (for detailed reviews see Raz, 2000; Raz et al., 2004; Raz and Rodrigue, 2006) as well as longitudinal studies (Resnick et al.,

2003). These results support the hypothesis of normal age-related GM decline being inversely related to the phylogenetic origin of each respective region, with younger structures being the last to mature as well as being more vulnerable to neurodegeneration (Terribilli et al., 2011; Toga et al., 2006). Recent magnetic resonance spectroscopy (MRS) studies provided evidence of specific age-related differences in neural viability and integrity, thus suggesting that the age-associated shrinkage in selected GM regions might reflect a decrease in the size and / or number of neurons (Kadota et al., 2001; Raz and Rodrigue, 2006).

Although WM volume was observed to remain relatively stable across adulthood, age appears to be the strongest predictor of differences in its microstructure (Kemper, 1994; Raz and Rodrigue, 2006), especially in white matter hyperintensities (WMH). WMHs were found to be caused by diverse neuropathological changes, including myelin pallor, atrophy of neuropil, damage in the subependymal ventricular linging (De Leeuw et al., 2001), subclinical ischemia (Pantoni et al., 1996), reduction in cerebral perfusion and greater vulnerability of the border zones (Brant-Zawadzki et al., 1987). Like in GM, the frontal regions appear to be affected first by WMH burden (Fazekas et al., 2005; Raz et al., 2003a,b,c). Furthermore, Artero et al. (2004) suggested a pattern of progression of WM lesions into temporal and occipital areas across time.

In summary, neuroanatomical aging is characterized by a widespread but well-ordered as well as region-specific brain tissue loss and CSF expansion.

1.2 Variability in brain aging

Though neuroanatomical aging is characterized by a widespread but rather specific pattern of alterations, multiple factors affect and modify those individual trajectories. For instance, several markers of poor health and / or an inappropriate lifestyle seem to be associated with the risk of cognitive decline, greater brain atrophy, and even dementia, including the metabolic syndrome, hypertension, diabetes, nicotine and alcohol abuse, elevated serum total homocysteine (tHcy), and lower levels of vitamin B12 (Chen et al., 2009; Clarke et al., 1998; Clarke, 2006; Clarke et al., 2007; Debette et al., 2010; Ellinson et al., 2004; Enzinger et al., 2005; Fitzpatrick et al., 2009; Middleton and Yafffe, 2009; Oulhaj et al., 2010; Solfrizzi et al., 2011; Steele et al., 2007; Zylberstein et al., 2011). Furthermore, combination of risk factors was found to further boost the risk (Luchsinger et al., 2005).

In contrast, a healthy and well-balanced lifestyle, including physical activity, normal body weight, smoking cessation, a Mediterranean diet, especially a high intake of unsaturated fatty acids, and moderate alcohol intake, was shown to lower the risk of cognitive decline and dementia (Erickson et al., 2010; Féart et al., 2010; Frisardi et al., 2010; Gu et al., 2010; Luchsinger and Gustafson, 2009; Nepal et al., 2010; Peters et al., 2008; Scarmeas et al., 2009; Solfrizzi et al., 2008; Xu et al., 2009).

In particular, hypertension appears to significantly boost the effects of aging on a wide range of neuroanatomical changes (De Leeuw et al., 2001; den Heijer et al., 2005; Carmelli et al., 1999; Goldstein et al., 2002; Raz et al., 2003a,b,c; Raz and Rodrigue, 2006; Salerno et al., 1992; Schmidt et al., 2003; Strassburger et al., 1997), even if treated (Raz et al., 2003a,b,c; van Swieten et al., 1991). Furthermore, hypertension was suggested to accelerate the age-related atrophy of the hippocampus (Du et al., 2006; Raz et al., 2005). Additionally, cardiovascular risk factors significantly accelerate age-related changes in GM, especially in the hippocampus and in posterior regions (Whalley et al., 2003; Williams et al., 2002). Hence, the hippocampus seems to be eminently vulnerable to those risk factors (Raz and Rodrigue, 2006).

Although age appears to be the strongest predictor of WMH, cerebrovascular risk factors were found to be additionally related to increased WMH burden (Raz and Rodrigue, 2006), including hypertension, ischemic attacks, atherosclerosis, decreased cortical blood vessel disease, and small vessel disease (Brown et al., 2002; De Leeuw et al., 2001; Kidwell et al., 2001; Markus et al., 2005; Moody et al., 2004; Pico et al., 2002). Moreover, the progression of WM lesions into temporal and occipital areas was observed to be associated with the presence of distinct clinical symptoms, including hypertension, depression, and poor cognitive functioning (Artero et al., 2004).

Furthermore, Apolipoprotein E (APOE) genotype was identified to be associated with faster cognitive decline in late life (Alexander et al., 2012; Donix et al., 2012; Harris and Deary, 2011; Van Gerven et al., 2012) as well as with the risk of developing cognitive impairment (Deary et al., 2002; Heise et al., 2011) and even AD (Rocchi et al., 2003; Trachtenberg et al., 2012). Especially the APOE ε4 allele is linked to the modification of cognitive functioning (Cosentino et al., 2008; Deary et al., 2002; Wishart et al., 2006) and GM reduction in healthy subjects (Bookheimer et al., 2000) as well as AD patients (Filippini et al., 2009).

1.3 Associations of brain structures with cognitive functions

To date, the associations between brain structure and cognitive functioning in normal aging are rather puzzling. Due to the lack of broad and well-controlled longitudinal studies combining neuroimaging with cognitive assessments, neither the true magnitude nor even the directions of age-related structure-function associations have been reliably assessed yet (Raz and Rodrigue, 2006).

Nevertheless, preliminary studies suggest better executive functioning to be associated with larger prefrontal cortices (Gunning-Dixon and Raz, 2003; Raz et al., 1998) as well as less frontal WMH (Gunning-Dixon and Raz, 2003). Enhanced skill acquisition performance was suggested to be associated with larger volumes of striatal structures, prefrontal cortex, and cerebellum (Kennedy and Raz, 2005; Raz, 2000; Woodruff-Pak et al., 2001). Longitudinal shrinkage of the entorhinal cortex (EC) was found to be related to reduced memory performance in healthy adults (Du et al., 2003; Rodrigue and Raz, 2004) and even future memory declines (de Leon et al., 2001). Decline in executive functioning was observed to be associated with longitudinal WMH increase (Cook et al., 2004).

On the other hand, several studies suggest that the degree of brain pathology does not directly relate to clinical manifestation of that damage (Fotenos et al., 2008; Katzman et al., 1989; Snowdon, 1997, 2003; Stern, 2006; Tyas et al., 2007). Higher premorbid IQ, education, occupational attainment, and participation in leisure activities were found to be associated with reduced risk of developing AD (Albert and Teresi, 1999; Alexander et al., 1997; Evans et al., 1993; Mortel et al., 1995; Stern et al., 1994, 1995; Stern, 2006; Richards and Sacker, 2003). Thus, the model of cognitive reserve (CR) was developed (Stern, 2002, 2003, 2006), suggesting that "the brain actively attempts to cope with brain damage by using preexisting cognitive processing approaches or by enlisting compensatory approaches. Individuals with more CR would be more successful at coping with the same amount of brain damage." (Stern, 2006). More specifically, Stern suggested two different – not mutually exclusive – mechanisms that could provide sustainment against structural brain damage before showing cognitive decline (Stern et al., 2005; Stern, 2006). Neural reserve refers to more efficient brain networks already existing in healthy individuals. Hence, these networks are less susceptible to disruption. Additionally, in neural compensation the disruption of preexisting networks is compensated by the use of alternate brain networks and cognitive strategies. Consequently, individuals who show the same level of cognitive decline or clinical severity may have divergent levels of underlying brain damage, with more advanced AD pathology being associated with higher levels of CR (Fotenos et al., 2008; Stern, 2006).

1.4 Accelerated brain atrophy in neurodegenerative diseases

With the growing number of studies that have investigated both normal and abnormal brain changes with age, most major neuropsychiatric and neurodegenerative disorders are now thought to arise due to deviations from normal structural brain aging, including schizophrenia (Giedd et al., 2009; Meda et al., 2008; Paus et al., 2008), depression (Paus et al., 2008), and AD (Ashburner et al., 2003).

Especially AD, the most common form of dementia (Brookmeyer et al., 2007), is widely assumed to be preceded by accelerated aging (for a controversial view see Nelson et al., 2011; Ohnishi et al., 2001). Recently, atrophic regions detected in AD patients were found to largely overlap with those regions showing a normal age-related decline in healthy control subjects (Dukart et al., 2011). The current understanding of the AD disease course

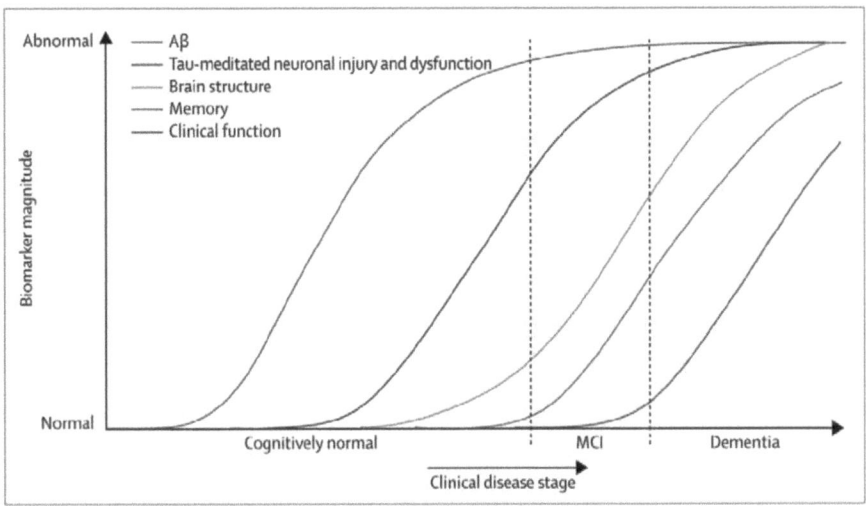

Figure 1.1: Dynamic biomarkers of the Alzheimer's pathological cascade. $A\beta$ is identified by CSF $A\beta_{42}$ or PET amlyloid imaging. Tau-mediated neuronal injury and dysfunction is identified by CSF tau or FDG-PET. Brain structure is measured using structural MRI. [Figure and legend from Jack et al. 2010.]

suggests that manifold pathological changes accumulate over many years in the first place years or decades before the onset of clinical symptoms; and secondly, cognitive decline occurs gradually, with dementia representing the final stage of the pathological cascade (Figure 1.1; Frisoni et al., 2010; Jack et al., 2010). These pathological changes include premature changes in gene expression (Cao et al., 2010; Saetre et al., 2011), accelerated age-associated changes of the default mode network (Jones et al., 2011), and most obviously, abnormal changes in brain structures at the stage of mild cognitive impairment (MCI; Driscoll et al., 2009; Spulber et al., 2010; Wang et al., 2009) and even in normal-functioning individuals (Clark et al., 2012; Davatzikos et al., 2009).

Particularly, the process of $A\beta$-plaque accumulation begins at least 5 – 10 years (Buchhave et al., 2012) or even up to two decades before probable manifestation of clinical symptoms and conversion to AD (Jack et al., 2009), but on its own is not sufficient to cause dementia (Aizenstein et al., 2008; Jack et al., 2010; Peskind et al., 2006; Price and Morris, 1999; Price et al., 2009; Savva et al., 2009). Especially low concentrations of CSF $A\beta_{42}$, associated with the formation of $A\beta$ plaques in the brain, were found to correlate with the clinical diagnosis of AD (Clark et al., 2003; Strozyk et al., 2003), but not with rates of brain atrophy (Josephs et al., 2008). At some point in the AD disease course accelerated neurodegeneration takes place, which is manifesting as atrophy, neuron loss, loss of synapses, and gliosis (Jack et al., 2010). Neurodegeneration, which precedes accelerated cognitive decline (Jack et al., 2010) as well as cognitive impairment (Buchhave et al., 2012; Shaw et al., 2009), is indicated by increasing CSF tau levels. However, increased phosphorylated tau (P-Tau) and total tau (T-Tau) is not specific for AD but seems to indicate neuronal injury and neurodegeneration in general (Jack et al., 2010; Hesse et al., 2001; Schoonenboom et al., 2012). Nevertheless, CSF tau was found to correlate with clinical disease severity, with increased levels being associated with greater cognitive impairment (Jack et al., 2010; Shaw et al., 2009). Although brain atrophy revealed by MRI in general is likewise not specific for AD, MRI was found to retain the closest relationship with cognitive decline (Jack et al., 2010; Vemuri et al., 2009a,b) suggesting a crucial role for structural MRI in predicting future conversion to AD (Jack et al., 2010; Frisoni et al., 2010). Importantly, the individual disease course is suggested to be modulated by diverse factors such as risk-associated and protective genes (e.g., APOE), converging comorbidity, and cognitive reserve (Figure 1.2; Ewers et al., 2011; Jack et al., 2010).

The myelin model of the human brain suggests an explanation of the anatomical processes underlying the continuum of cognitive decline in later life leading to AD and integrates the diverse results regarding the pathogenesis of AD (Bartzokis, 2004, 2011; Bartzokis et al., 2012; Lu et al., 2011, 2013). It proposes that the processes of myelin development, maintenance, and the eventual breakdown of the myelin repair process across the lifespan are underlying the unique cognitive abilities in humans, but are also underlying the unique vulnerability to neuropsychiatric (e.g. schizophrenia) and neurodegenerative disorders such as AD (Bartzokis, 2004, 2011). More specifically, the model assumes regions that myelinate later in brain development, are first and maximally affected by the aging process (Bartzokis, 2004, 2011; Lu et al., 2013). Likewise, the pattern of AD lesions was suggested to recapitulate the myelination pattern in reverse (Braak and Braak, 1996), with the earliest maturing cortex being least vulnerable to aging and AD (Figure 1.3; Ewers et al., 2011; Gogtay et al., 2004).

In particular, the need for myelin repair increases in older age and is most distinct in later-myelinating regions (e.g., frontal lobe white matter, genu of the corpus callosum) due to higher proportions of thinly-myelinated axons in these regions (Bartzokis, 2004, 2011; Lu et al., 2013; Marner et al., 2003;

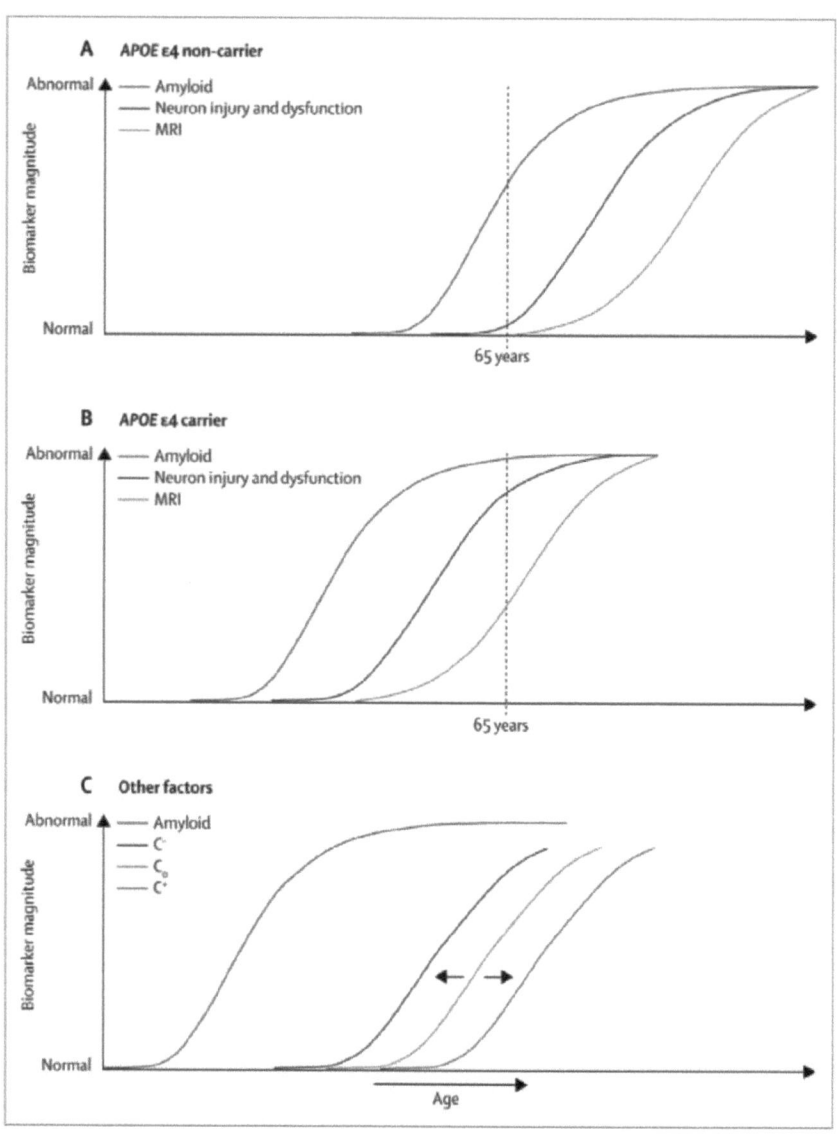

Figure 1.2: Modulators of biomarker temporal relationships. (A,B) Relative to a fixed age (here, 65 years), the hypothesized effect of APOE ε4 is to shift β-amyloid plaque deposition and the neurodegenerative cascade both to an earlier age compared with ε4 non-carriers. **(C)** The hypothesized effect of the presence of different diseases and genes on cognition: C^- = cognition in the presence of comorbidities (e.g., Lewy bodies or vascular disease) or risk amplification genes; C^+ = cognition in patients with enhanced cognitive reserve or protective genes; C_0 = cognition in individuals without comorbidity or enhanced cognitive reserve. [Figure and legend from Jack et al. 2010.]

Salat et al., 2005). Contrariwise, successful demyelination slows with age (Bartzokis, 2011; Shen et al., 2008; Shields et al., 1999). Thus, as a function of genetic variability and several other modifying factors (see section 1.2), the myelin repair processes become less efficient and effective, resulting in age-related myelin breakdown and thus in axonal transport disruptions. As a by-product, Aβ is suggested to be released and bound to the receptors, which may increase toxicity to synapses (Bartzokis, 2011; Laurén et al., 2009; Selkoe, 2008; Shankar et al., 2008), surrounding myelin (Bartzokis, 2011; Muse et al., 2001), and dendrites (Bartzokis, 2011). Likewise, an increase in hyperphosphorylated tau is also proposed to represent a byproduct of the myelin repair process (Bartzokis, 2011). Finally, the age-related myelin breakdown results in an "Alzheimerization" of the human brain, including Aβ-

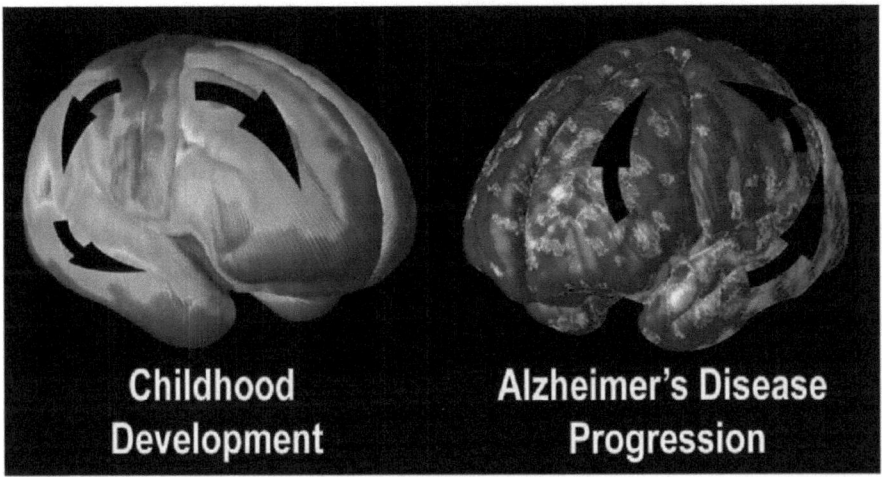

Childhood Development

Alzheimer's Disease Progression

Figure 1.3: **Degenerative sequence of brain changes in AD is the reverse order of the normal developmental sequence.** In a process termed retrogenesis (e.g., by Reisberg et al., 1999), cortical regions that mature earliest in infancy tend to degenerate last in AD. The developmental sequence echoes the phylogenetic sequence in which structures evolved. The most heavily myelinated structures, with least neuronal plasticity, resist AD-related neurodegeneration. Arrows denote the childhood cortical maturation sequence (*left panel;* Gogtay et al., 2004) and the gray matter atrophy sequence in AD (*right panel;* Thompson et al., 2003). Images are from time-lapse films compiled from cortical models in subjects scanned longitudinally with MRI. [Figure and legend from Ewers et al. 2011.]

plaque accumulation and increasing CSF tau levels, as well as synapse and neuron loss, leading to distinct brain lesions (Bartzokis, 2011). Consequently, aging – and more specifically, brain aging – is associated with a widespread and sequential pattern of tissue loss, whereas early and / or more pronounced myelin breakdown may lead to severe pathologic manifestations of diseases such as AD.

1.5 The *BrainAGE* approach

Relying upon previously acquired insights and models, accelerated and thus pathological brain atrophy should be recognizable quite early and before the onset of cognitive decline and clinical symptoms. Hence, identifying accelerated brain atrophy before the onset of clinical symptoms as well as predicting the prospective cognitive decline and subsequent transition to AD will contribute to early treatment or prophylaxis.

Assuming AD to be preceded by precocious and / or accelerated brain aging (Bartzokis, 2011; Driscoll et al., 2009; Spulber et al., 2010), a straightforward and efficient solution is to model healthy aging on the one hand, and to identify accelerated (thus pathological) brain atrophy on the other. Consequently, in order to recognize faster brain atrophy, a model of healthy and normal brain aging is needed. A straightforward and efficient solution is to model age regression based on normal brain anatomy, such that an individual's age can be accurately estimated from his / her brain scan alone.

The *BrainAGE* approach takes into account the widespread, sequential brain tissue loss associated with aging. Based on single time-point structural MRI, the complex, multidimensional aging patterns across the whole brain are aggregated to one single value, i.e. the estimated brain age (Figure 1.4A). Consequently, although using only one MRI scan per subject, the deviation in brain atrophy from normal brain aging can be directly quantified (Figure 1.4B).

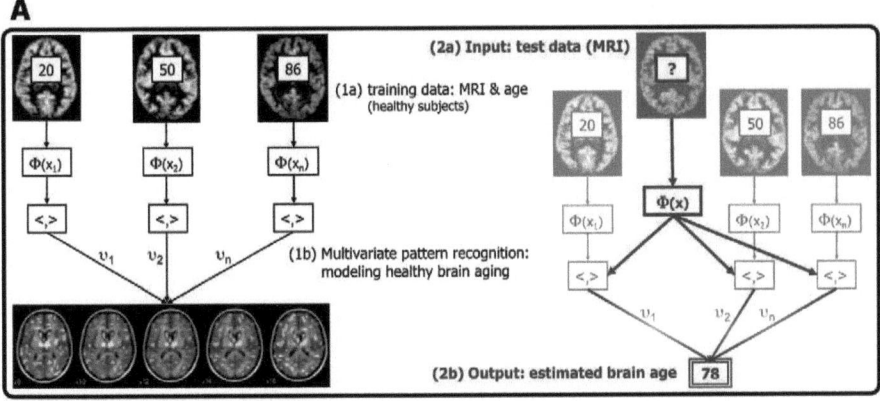

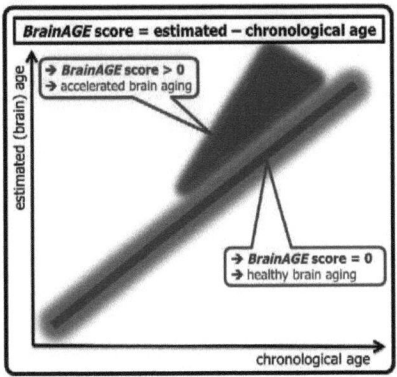

Figure 1.4: Depiction of the *BrainAGE* concept. (A) The model of healthy brain aging is trained with the chronological age and preprocessed structural MRI data of a training sample (*left;* with an exemplary illustration of the most important voxel locations that were used by the age regression model). Subsequently, the individual brain ages of previously unseen test subjects are estimated, based on their MRI data (picture modified from Schölkopf and Smola, 2002). **(B)** The difference between the estimated and chronological age results in the *BrainAGE* score. Consequently, positive *BrainAGE* scores indicate accelerated brain aging. [Figure and legend modified from Franke et al. 2012a.]

In **chapter 2**, the *BrainAGE* framework, which automatically estimates the age of healthy subjects from their T1-weighted MRI scans, is introduced and tested. In **chapter 3**, the stability of individual *BrainAGE* scores over multiple time points and across different scanners is examined. Furthermore, the *BrainAGE* framework is implemented to examine longitudinal brain changes in cognitively healthy subjects, subjects with MCI, and AD patients. In **chapter 4**, the effects of type 2 diabetes mellitus (T2DM) on individual brain aging as well as its relationships to clinically significant risk factors and functionality measures is investigated. In **chapter 5**, the *BrainAGE* approach is implemented to predict prospective conversion to AD on an individual subject level.

Chapter 2.

Estimating the age of healthy subjects from T1-weighted MRI scans using kernel methods: Exploring the influence of various parameters [1]

2.1 Abstract

The early identification of brain anatomy deviating from the normal pattern of growth and atrophy, such as in Alzheimer's disease (AD), has the potential to improve clinical outcomes through early intervention. Recently, Davatzikos et al. (2009) supported the hypothesis that pathologic atrophy in AD is an accelerated aging process, implying accelerated brain atrophy. In order to recognize faster brain atrophy, a model of healthy brain aging is needed first. Here, we introduce a framework for automatically and efficiently estimating the age of healthy subjects from their T1-weighted MRI scans using a kernel method for regression. This method was tested on over 650 healthy subjects, aged 19 86 years, and collected from four different scanners. Furthermore, the influence of various parameters on estimation accuracy was analyzed. Our age estimation framework included automatic preprocessing of the T1-weighted images, dimension reduction via principal component analysis, training of a relevance vector machine (RVM; Tipping, 2000) for regression, and finally estimating the age of the subjects from the test samples. The framework proved to be a reliable, scanner-independent, and efficient method for age estimation in healthy subjects, yielding a correlation of $r = 0.92$ between the estimated and the real age in the test samples and a mean absolute error of 5 years. The results indicated favorable performance of the RVM and identified the number of training samples as the critical factor for prediction accuracy. Ap-

---

[1] Research article [published as: Franke, K., Ziegler, G., Klöppel, S., Gaser, C., and Alzheimer's Disease Neuroimaging Initiative (2010). Estimating the age of healthy subjects from T1-weighted MRI scans using kernel methods: exploring the influence of various parameters. *Neuroimage*, 50(3):883–892.]

plying the framework to people with mild AD resulted in a mean *"Brain Age Gap Estimation"* (*BrainAGE*) score of +10 years.

2.2 Introduction

During the normal aging process, the brain changes due to progressive (e.g., cell growth and myelination) and regressive neuronal processes (e.g., cell death and atrophy). Brain development and healthy aging have been found to follow a specific pattern. Using a semiautomated approach based on a very crude geometrical method for the segmentation of the MRI data, Pfefferbaum et al. (1994) showed that gray matter (GM) volume increases from birth until the age of four and thereafter decreases continuously until subjects reach their 70's. White matter (WM) volume increases steadily until around the age of 20 when it plateaus. Cerebrospinal fluid (CSF) exhibits a complementary pattern, remaining constant until about 20 years of age and increasing steadily thereafter (Pfefferbaum et al., 1994). A similar, but more recent study conducted a fully automated voxel-based morphometry (VBM) study with 465 normal subjects aged 17 – 79 years to explore global and regional effects of age (Good et al., 2001). The results of this cross-sectional VBM study also suggested a linear decline in GM to be predominant in normal aging as well as a linear increase of CSF with age. Furthermore, local areas of accelerated GM decline and microstructural changes in WM were reported, suggesting a heterogeneous and complex pattern of atrophy across the adult life span (Good et al., 2001). Evidence for a region-specific and non-linear pattern of neurodegenerative age-related changes in GM volume was also provided by cross-sectional morphometric analyses (Terribilli et al., 2011) as well as longitudinal data comparison (Resnick et al., 2003). These results support the hypothesis of normal age-related GM decline being inversely related to the phylogenetic origin of each respective region, with younger structures being the last to mature as well as being more vulnerable to neurodegeneration (see also Terribilli et al., 2011; Toga et al., 2006).

Diseases such as Alzheimer's disease (AD) or schizophrenia alter brain structures in diverse and abnormal modes (Ashburner et al., 2003; Meda et al., 2008). Developing a fully automated, reliable, and sufficiently sensitive as well as specific method for the early identification of such pathologic brain developments even before the onset of clinical symptoms has been given great emphasis during the last years (Ashburner, 2009; Davatzikos et al., 2009). Pathologic brain development patterns have been explored and subsequently a variety of classification methods have been employed to separate one or more groups of patients from healthy controls (Davatzikos et al., 2005, 2008a,b; Fan et al., 2008a,b; Klöppel et al., 2008a,b, 2009; Liu et al., 2004; Teipel et al., 2007; Vemuri et al., 2008, 2009a,b). Most of these studies used a processing sequence that started with segmenting and spatially normalizing MRI data, then applied some kind of feature selection or dimensionality reduction, e.g., principal component analysis (PCA), trained a classifier based on Support Vector Machines (SVM), and finally estimated the classification accuracy with (jackknife) cross-validation. Typically, the sample sizes of these classification studies were rather small, thus entailing the risk of overfitting, which could potentially produce considerable underperformance of the trained classifier when it is applied to a completely new sample. In order to increase sensitivity and reliability of the classification methods, Ashburner (2009) advocated the initiation and usage of multi-scanner data sets tracking a large number of subjects. Integrating data from different scanners in a linear SVM classification study, Klöppel et al. (2008b) reported rates for correctly classified AD patients versus healthy controls of around 90%. This suggests that kernel methods like SVM have the capability to generalize on data obtained from various scanners.

Recently, Davatzikos et al. (2009) showed the longitudinal progression of AD-like patterns in brain atrophy in the normal aging subjects and furthermore an accelerated AD-like atrophy in subjects with mild cognitive impairment (MCI). These results support the hypothesis of AD being a form of accelerated aging, implying accelerated brain atrophy (Driscoll et al., 2009; Fotenos et al., 2008; Sluimer et al., 2009; Spulber et al., 2010; Wang et al., 2009; for a controversial view, see Ohnishi et al., 2001). In case of schizophrenia, a similar hypothesis of the disease being a syndrome of accelerated aging has been presented (Kirkpatrick et al., 2008). If these hypotheses hold true in future research, accelerated and thus pathologic brain atrophy should be recognizable quite early and before the onset of clinical symptoms. In order to recognize faster brain atrophy, a model of healthy and normal brain aging is needed. A straightforward and efficient solution is to model age regression based on normal brain anatomy such that an individual's age can be accurately estimated from its brain scan alone.

Until recently, only a few studies were published that perform age estimation or prediction based on MRI scans. Lao et al. (2004) tested an SVM-based classification method by assigning their elderly subjects into one of four age groups and reached an accuracy rate of 90%. In order to demonstrate the performance of his algorithm for diffeomorphic image registration, Ashburner (2007) estimated the age of subjects based on their brain images utilizing a relevance vector machine (RVM) for regression (Tipping, 2000, 2001). As a measure for prediction accuracy, a root mean squared error (RMSE) of 6.5 years was reported. Another method used quantitative brain water maps to predict age and gender of 44 healthy volunteers aged 23 – 74 years (Neeb et al., 2006). A linear discriminant analysis with jackknife cross-validation for age prediction resulted in a median absolute deviation between real and predicted age of ± 6.3 years.

Although a number of approaches exist that model the pattern of healthy neuronal aging using MRI data, to our knowledge neither the influences of different processing parameters on age estimation were explored, nor was it used for early detection of abnormal aging processes. Large discrepancies between the true and estimated age could indicate pathologic structural changes. Therefore, this work could help to contribute to an early diagnosis and better understanding of neurodegenerative diseases as well as to a more specific and earlier intervention.

In this paper, we present a framework for automatically and efficiently estimating the age of healthy subjects from T1-weighted MRI scans using RVM-based regression. To avoid overfitting as well as to increase sensitivity and reliability, we combine data from the IXI database and a second sample (Gaser et al., 1999). In total, data from over 650 healthy subjects aged between 19 – 86 years, collected from four different scanners, were included. To explore the influence of various parameters on the age estimation framework, several analyses on this large database were conducted. We sought to identify the optimal set of processing parameters when the age of data coming from a new scanner had to be estimated. Another goal of this study was a comparison of the performance of well-established SVM with RVM-based regression. SVM require the optimization of a number of parameters (described in more detail in 2.2.4). We therefore expect RVM to be more stable and less vulnerable to parameter selection errors than SVM. Due to the "curse of dimensionality", we expect the age estimation to be more accurate if the dimensionality of the preprocessed data is reduced by a dimension reduction method like PCA.

Finally, the age estimation framework will be applied to a clinical sample from the Alzheimer's Disease Neuroimaging Initiative (ADNI) database, which includes T1-weighted images of people with mild AD as well as healthy elderly control subjects. Compared to the group of healthy subjects, we hypothesized that the AD group would have a systematically larger gap between the estimated brain age and the true age due to accelerated brain aging that is presumed to be responsible for the diseased state.

2.3 Methods
2.3.1 Subjects / database

To train and test the age estimation framework with respect to prediction accuracy and reliability, we used brain MR images of healthy subjects from the publicly accessible IXI database[2] and from our own sample. In February 2009, the IXI database contained T1-images from 550 normal subjects aged 19 – 86 years, which were collected on three different scanners (Philips 1.5T, General Electric 1.5T, Philips 3T). The subjects were pseudo-randomly split into a training sample, which was used to generate the regression models in relevance vector regression (RVR) and support vector regression (SVR), and a test sample: after sorting the subjects by age, every fourth subject entered the test sample. Since three subjects, for whom no age was given, had to be excluded, the training sample *"TRAIN1–3"* consisted of 410 subjects, and the first test sample (*"TEST1–3"*) consisted of the remaining 137 subjects from the IXI database, acquired on the three different scanners mentioned above. The second test sample (*"TEST4"*) originally served as a control group in a clinical study (Gaser et al., 1999). TEST4 contained T1-images from 108 healthy subjects aged 20 – 59 years, which were obtained on a fourth scanner (Philips 1.5T).

The characteristics of the three groups are given in Table 2.1, and the distribution of age within the training sample and both test samples are shown in Figure 2.1.

---

[2] www.brain-development.org

Table 2.1: Characteristics of the subjects in the training groups (TRAIN1-3) and both test samples (TEST1-3 and TEST4). TRAIN1-3 and TEST1-3 were collected from the IXI database utilizing three different scanners, whereas the MRI data of the TEST4 sample were collected on a fourth scanner and were not used for training.

	IXI database (scanner 1-3)		Own sample (scanner 4)
	TRAIN1-3	TEST1-3	TEST4
No. subjects	410	137	108
Males / Females	184 / 226	58 / 79	68 / 40
Age mean (SD)	48.2 (16.6)	48.0 (16.7)	32.2 (10.0)
Age range	20 – 86	19 – 83	20 – 59

2.3.2 Preprocessing of structural MRI data

Preprocessing of the images was done using the SPM8 package[3] and the VBM8 toolbox[4]. All T1-weighted images were corrected for bias-field inhomogeneities, then spatially normalized and segmented into GM, WM, and CSF within the same generative model (Ashburner and Friston, 2005). The segmentation procedure was further extended by accounting for partial volume effects (Tohka et al., 2004), by applying adaptive maximum a posteriori estimations (Rajapakse et al., 1997), and by applying hidden Markov random field model (Cuadra et al., 2005) as described by Gaser (2009). Only GM images were used for the TRAIN1-3 sample and to test the age estimation model. To make this age estimation framework fast and efficient, the images were additionally processed with affne registration (AF) and smoothed with an 8 mm full-width-at-half-maximum (FWHM) smoothing kernel (S8). In order to reduce data size the spatial resolution was set to 8 mm (R8), resulting an image size of about 3700 voxels per subject.

Furthermore – for comparison – the images were registered non-linearly (NL), a 4 mm FWHM smoothing kernel (S4) was used, and spatial resolution

---

[3] www.fil.ion.ucl.ac.uk/spm
[4] http://dbm.neuro.uni-jena.de

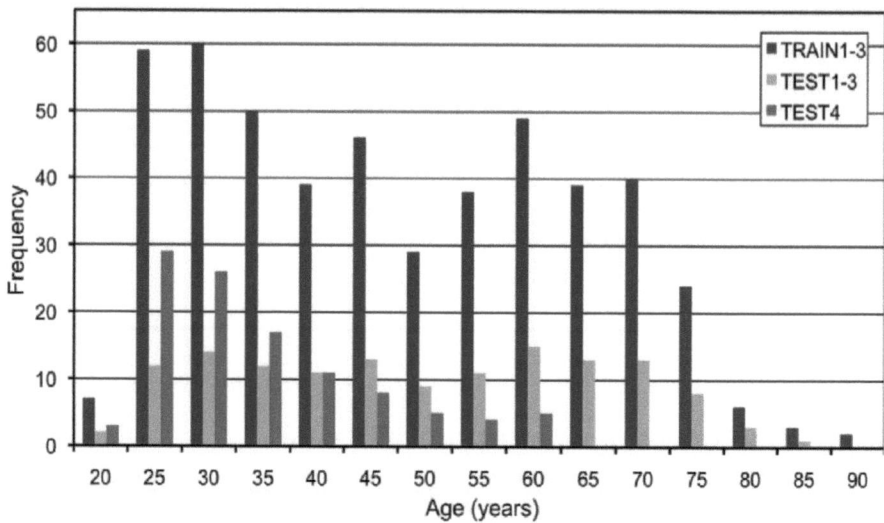

Figure 2.1: Shown is the age distribution within our training group (TRAIN1-3) and both test samples (TEST1-3 and TEST4). TRAIN1-3 and TEST1-3 were collected from the IXI database utilizing three different scanners, whereas the MRI data of TEST4 were collected on a different scanner (not used for training). [Figure and legend modified from Franke et al. 2010.]

was set to 3 mm (R3) and 4 mm (R4). As non-linear spatial normalization, the approach implemented in the new "Segment toolbox" in SPM8 was used.

2.3.3 Data reduction

Usually, there are high spatial correlations in voxel-based structural images, which probably lead to redundant voxels. Moreover, not every single voxel is equally relevant for age prediction. Because of that and due to the "curse of dimensionality", data reduction or feature selection might be necessary to obtain meaningful results from the pattern recognition analysis (Ashburner, 2009; Duchesnay et al., 2007; Guyon and Elisseeff, 2003). Commonly, PCA is conducted to reduce the dimensionality of the data.

Using the "MATLAB Toolbox for Dimensionality Reduction" (version 0.7b; van der Maaten, 2007, 2008), PCA was applied to the preprocessed images of the training sample. Then the two test samples were reduced using the resulting PCA transformation. Corresponding to the number of subjects in the training sample, the data finally had a size of 410 principal components per subject.

2.3.4 Support vector regression (SVR)

The main idea behind SVMs is the transformation of training data from input space into high-dimensional space – the feature space – via a mapping function Φ (Bennett and Campbell, 2003; Schölkopf and Smola, 2002). For the purpose of classification, the hyperplane that best separates the groups is computed within this feature space, resulting in a non-linear decision boundary within the input space. The best separating hyperplane is found by maximizing the margin between the two groups. The data points lying on the margin boundaries are called support vectors since only these are used to specify the optimal separating hyperplane. In the case of overlapping class distributions, some training data points are allowed to be misclassified, resulting in some support vectors lying within the margin or on the wrong side of the margin boundary (soft-margin classification; Bishop, 2006).

For the case of real-valued output functions (rather than just binary outputs as used in classification), the SV algorithm was generalized to regression estimation (Bennett and Campbell, 2003; Schölkopf and Smola, 2002). In SVR, a function has to be found that fits as many data points as possible. Analogous to the soft margin in classification, the regression line is surrounded by a tube. Data points lying within that tube do not influence the course of the regression line. Data points lying on the edge or outside that tube are called support vectors (Figure 2.2A). The expansion of the tube can be determined in a variety of ways, with ε-SVR and ν-SVR being the most common approaches. In ε-SVR, the a priori specified constant ε defines the width of the linear ε-insensitive tube around the regression line. Data points falling within this ε-insensitive tube are not penalized, and are therefore not

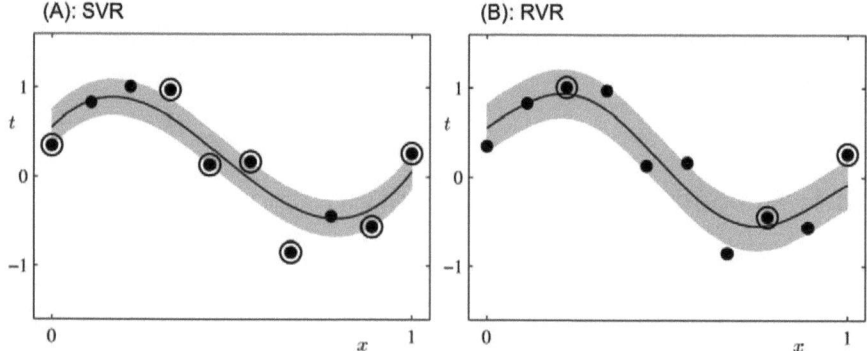

Figure 2.2: Illustration of **(A)** SVR and **(B)** RVR (modified from Bishop, 2006). Data points are shown as black dots; circles indicate **(A)** support vectors and **(B)** relevance vectors, respectively. [Figure and legend modified from Franke et al. 2010.]

taken as support vectors. In ν-SVR, the a priori specified sparsity parameter ν defines the upper bound on the fraction of support vectors, i.e., data points lying outside an ε-insensitive tube that is automatically adjusted in width. To control the behavior of ε-SVR and ν-SVR, the type of kernel has to be chosen, along with two more parameters: C, which controls for model complexity, and ε or ν, respectively. A short overview of SVM can be found in Bennett and Campbell (2003). More details can be found in Bishop (2006) or Schölkopf and Smola (2002).

2.3.5 Relevance vector regression (RVR)

RVMs were introduced by Tipping (2000) as a Bayesian alternative to SVMs for obtaining sparse solutions to pattern recognition tasks. Moreover, they do not suffer from some limitations of the SVM as their predictions are being probabilistic rather than binary and do not need the determination of additional parameters. In contrast to the support vectors in SVM, the relevance vectors in RVM appear to represent the prototypical examples within the specified classification or regression task instead of solely representing separating attributes.

Furthermore severe overfitting associated with the maximum likelihood estimation of the model parameters was avoided by imposing an explicit zero-mean Gaussian prior (Ghosh and Mujumdar, 2008; Zheng et al., 2008). This prior is a characteristic feature of the RVM, and its use results in a vector of independent hyperparameters that reduces the data set (Faul and Tipping, 2002; Tipping and Faul, 2003; Tipping, 2000). Therefore, in most cases the number of relevance vectors is much smaller than the number of support vectors (Figure 2.2B).

To control the behavior of the RVR, only the type of kernel has to be chosen. All other parameters are automatically estimated by the learning procedure itself. More details can be found in Bishop (2006), Schölkopf and Smola (2002), or Tipping (2000, 2001).

2.3.6 Computing the age estimation model

We used the freely available toolbox "The Spider" (Version 1.71; Weston et al., 2006) running under MATLAB 7.4.0 to compute the final age regression model.

The T1-weighted MRI data of the training sample TRAIN1-3 and both test samples TEST1-3 and TEST4 were preprocessed by applying affine registration, followed by smoothing with an FWHM kernel of 8 mm and resampling with spatial resolution of 8 mm (AF_S8_R8). The pre-processed data were reduced using PCA, and the RVR age estimation model was trained using this reduced data set. The type of kernel was set to be a polynomial of degree 1, due to its fast convergence rate. We also tested the performance of non-linear kernels. Age estimation did not improve (results not shown), despite adding at least one more parameter (e.g., kernel width). Finally, the ages of the subjects in TEST1–3 and TEST4 were estimated (Figure 2.3, box ①).

To measure the accuracy of the age estimations, we used the mean absolute error:

MAE = $1/n * \Sigma_i |g_i' - g_i|$, (2.1)

with n being the number of subjects in the test sample, g_i the real age, and g_i' the age estimated by the regression model. We found MAE to be the most meaningful measure for assessing the influence of different parameters. For comparison, the root mean squared error:

RMSE = $[1/n * \Sigma_i (g_i' - g_i)^2]^{1/2}$, (2.2)

as well as the correlation coefficient were calculated. Because of the restricted age range in the sample TEST4 and a resulting underestimation of the correlations between the real age and the predicted age, the correlations were corrected following Holmes (1990).

2.3.7 Systematic analyses of different parameters influencing the age estimation model

We first compared the age estimation accuracies when testing the age estimation model with data from "known" scanners (i.e., TEST1–3) versus when testing with data from a "new" scanner (i.e., TEST4; Figure 2.3, box ①).

Secondly, in order to explore the ability to generalize across scanners, we included data from the fourth scanner into the training sample (Figure 2.3, box ②). To test for the effect of scanners on prediction accuracy, the whole IXI data set as well as TEST4 was randomly and separately split into four groups. This resulted in a training set that included 410 randomly selected subjects from scanners 1–3 (IXI) plus 81 randomly selected subjects from scanner 4, and a test set including the remaining 137 subjects from the IXI sample as well as the remaining 27 subjects from scanner 4. The age estimation framework was trained two times: In the first run, the RVR was trained with 410 randomly selected subjects from the IXI sample (scanners 1–3) only. Then the age of the remaining 137 subjects from the IXI sample and of the 27 randomly selected subjects of TEST4 was estimated. In the second run, the RVR was trained with the same 410 IXI subjects as in the first training run plus the randomly selected training sample from TEST4. Again, age was estimated for the actual test subjects from all four scanners. After repeating the whole procedure 20 times, the results were averaged over the trials.

Thirdly, the influence of data reduction and different kernel regression methods was tested (Figure 2.3, box ③). For comparison, the age estimation model was also computed using ε-SVR and ν-SVR. As before, a polynomial kernel of degree 1 was chosen. Here, the cost parameter C and the width of the ε-tube or ν for ε-SVR and ν-SVR, respectively, also have to be set. Instead of performing an exhaustive grid search and cross-validation to find these model parameters, we followed Cherkassky and Ma (2004) in choosing the size of the ε-SVR parameters, resulting in $C = 98$ and $\varepsilon = 0.064$. With respect to ν-SVR, we followed Chalimourda et al. (2004), resulting in $C = 20500$ and $\nu = 0.54$. Furthermore, we also used the default values of the toolbox with $C = 1$, $\varepsilon = 0.1$, and $\nu = 0.5$, respectively.

Fourthly, to explore which type of preprocessing is best for age prediction, we varied three parameters during preprocessing: (i) affine (AF) vs. non-linear (NL) registration, (ii) 4 mm (S4) vs. 8 mm (S8) FWHM smoothing kernel, and (iii) 3 mm (R3), 4 mm (R4) vs. 8 mm (R8) for spatial resolution. Memory demands forbade spatial resolutions below 3 mm with this very large subject pool (Figure 2.3, box ④).

Fifthly, we analyzed the influence of the size of the training data set (i.e., the number of subjects), comparing the full training sample ("*1/1 TRAIN1–3*") against half of the original training sample ("*1/2 TRAIN1–3*") and against a quarter of the original training sample ("*1/4 TRAIN1–3*") (Figure 2.3, box ⑤).

Finally, all the parameter variations examined before were integrated into

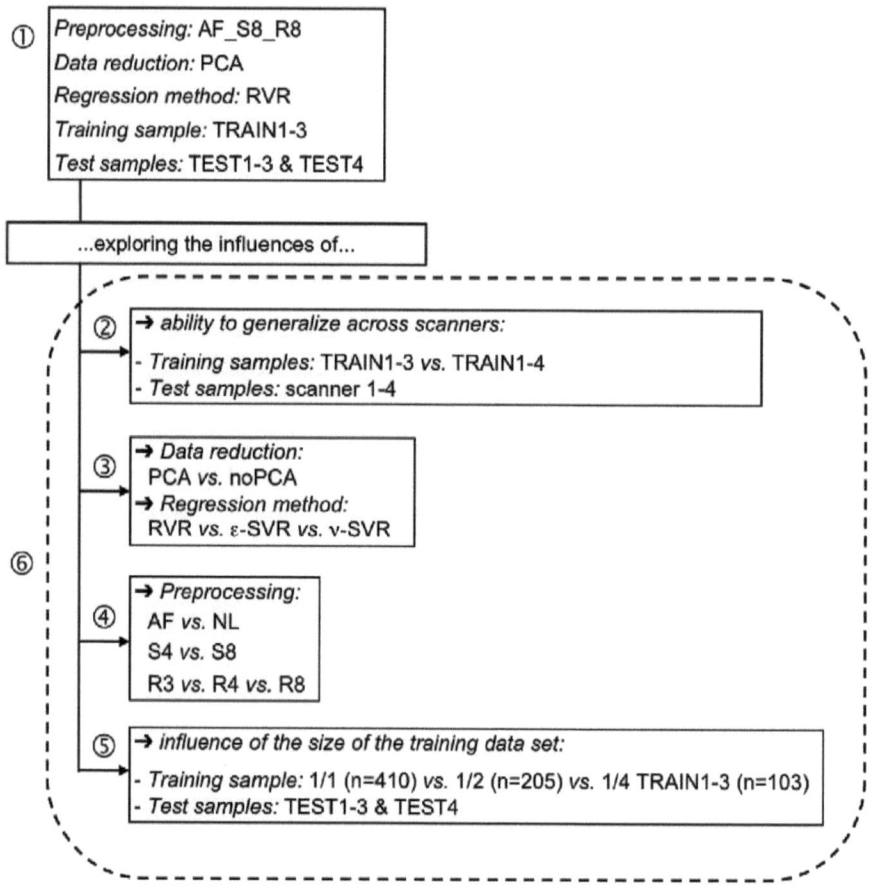

Figure 2.3: Shown is an overview of the six analyses conducted within this age estimation study to explore the influences of various parameters on age estimation accuracy. [Figure and legend from Franke et al. 2010.]
[*Abbreviations:* AF, affine registration; NL, non-linear registration; S4/S8, smoothing kernel = 4 mm/8 mm; R3/R4/R8, spatial resolution = 3 mm/4 mm/8 mm; PCA, principal component analysis; TRAIN1–3, training sample; TEST1–3 and TEST4, test samples; RVR, relevance vector regression; SVR, support vector regression]

one analysis to assess the proportional amount of influence of each parameter considered (Figure 2.3, box ⑥).

2.3.8 Application of the age estimation framework to data from the ADNI database

To test the potential of this age estimation framework to provide clinically relevant predictions, the age of people with early AD and cognitively normal elderly control subjects was estimated. This test sample incorporated MRI data obtained from the Alzheimer's Disease Neuroimaging Initiative (ADNI) database[5]. The ADNI was launched in 2003 by the National Institute on Aging (NIA), the National Institute of Biomedical Imaging and Bioengineering (NIBIB), the Food and Drug Administration (FDA), private pharmaceutical companies, and non-profit organizations as a $60 million, 5-year public-private partnership. The primary goal of ADNI has been to test whether serial magnetic resonance imaging (MRI), positron emission tomography (PET), other biological markers, and clinical and neuropsychological assessment can be combined to measure the progression of mild cognitive impairment (MCI) and early Alzheimer's disease (AD). Determination of sensitive and specific markers of very early AD progression is intended to aid researchers and clinicians to develop new treatments and monitor their effectiveness as well as to lessen the time and cost of clinical trials. The Principle Investigator of this initiative is Michael W. Weiner, M.D., VA Medical Center and University of California, San Francisco. ADNI is the result of efforts of many co-investigators from a broad range of academic institutions and private corporations, and subjects have been recruited from over 50 sites across the U.S. and Canada. The initial goal of ADNI was to recruit 800 adults, ages 55 to 90 years, to participate in the research – approximately 200 cognitively normal older individuals to be followed for 3 years, 400 people with MCI to be fol-

---

[5] www.loni.ucla.edu/ADNI

lowed for 3 years, and 200 people with early AD to be followed for 2 years. For up-to-date information, see www.adni-info.org.

To compare the age estimations of people with early AD and cognitively normal elderly subjects, two groups were formed and analyzed using the age estimation framework. The AD group included T1-weighted images of subjects who had a global Clinical Dementia Rating Scale (CDR; Morris, 1993) score of 1 at baseline (n = 102; mean Mini-Mental State Examination score = 22.9 (MMSE; Cockrell and Folstein, 1988)). Similarly, the group of healthy controls (NO) included T1-weighted images of subjects who had a global CDR score of 0 at baseline (n = 232; mean MMSE score = 29.1). Detailed characteristics of both groups can also be found in Table 2.2.

In order to get a meaningful comparative deviation score, the difference (or gap) between the estimated and the true age was computed. This deviation is termed *"Brain Age Gap Estimation"* (*BrainAGE*) score. The mean *BrainAGE* of the NO group should consequently be zero.

2.4 Results
2.4.1 Performance measures

The age of healthy subjects in both test samples was accurately estimated from their MRI scans (Table 2.3), with an overall correlation of r = 0.92 and an MAE of just 5 years. The age prediction tended to be slightly more accurate

Table 2.2: Characteristics of the two groups from the ADNI database used in the application of the age estimation framework (AD and NO).

	ADNI database	
	AD (CDR = 1)	NO (CDR = 0)
No. subjects	102	232
Males / Females	47 / 55	119 / 113
Age mean (SD)	75.8 (8.2)	76.0 (5.1)
Age range	55 – 88	60 – 90

Table 2.3: Performance measures of the age estimation model for TEST1–3 and TEST4. Results indicate that the age of the healthy subjects in both test samples could be accurately estimated from MRI scans.

	TEST1–3	TEST4	TEST1–3 + TEST4
Mean absolute error (MAE)	4.61	5.44	4.98
Root mean squared error (RMSE)	5.90	6.73	6.28
Correlation (r)	0.94	0.89	0.92
Confidence interval (at overall mean age of 41 years)	± 10.7	± 11.7	± 11.5

in TEST1–3, which consisted of subjects scanned on the same three scanners as the subjects in the training sample, whereas the subjects in TEST4 had been scanned on a scanner that was not included in the training sample. The 95% confidence interval for the prediction of age was stable along the age range, with no broadening at old age (cf. age = 20 ± 11.6 years, age = 80 ± 11.7 years; Figure 2.4). Furthermore, a correlation of $r = -0.015$ between MAE and the true age indicated no systematical bias in the age estimations as a function of true ages.

The results did not depend on gender in terms of MAE (5.04 years for male, 4.92 years for female subjects) or correlation ($r = 0.92$ for both genders). Again, there was no correlation between estimation accuracy and true age for either gender (male: $r = 0.03$; female: $r = -0.05$). The most important features in the MRI data that were used by the RVR for estimating the age are shown in Figure 2.5.

2.4.2 Influence of different scanners

As shown in the first analysis, estimating the age from MRI scans after training an RVR yields highly accurate predictions, even for completely new data from another scanner. To analyze the influence of scanners on the accuracy of age estimation, the analysis described in section 2.2.7 was conducted, in which 75% of the subjects from either scanners 1–3 only or all scanners were

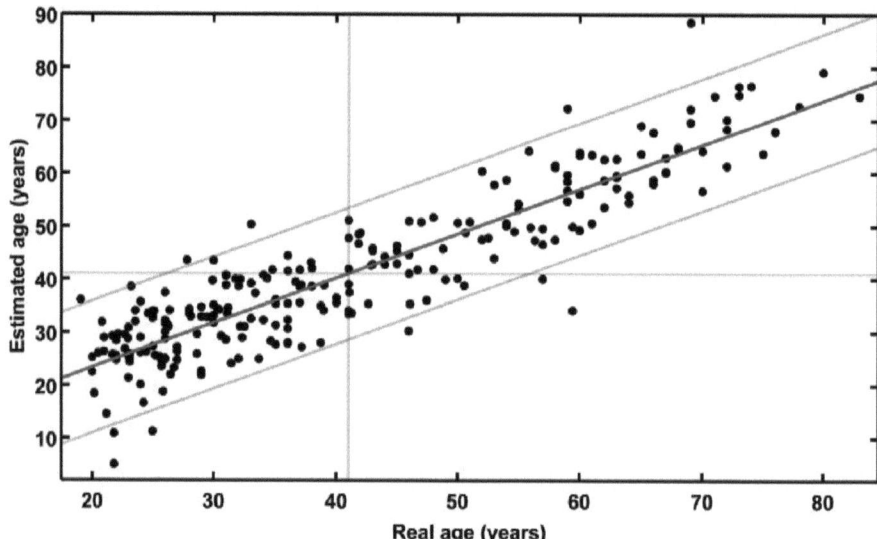

Figure 2.4: Estimated age and real age are shown for the whole test sample (TEST1–3 + TEST4) with the confidence interval (light red lines) at a real age of 41 years of ± 11.5 years. The overall correlation between estimated and real age is $r = 0.92$, and the overall MAE = 4.98 years. [Figure and legend modified from Franke et al. 2010.]

used as the training group. After averaging the results from 20 trials, no difference in estimation accuracy was found between both training runs. When analyzing scanners separately, the accuracy of age prediction varied only slightly between individual scanners (Figure 2.6).

2.4.3 Impact of regression methods and data reduction

Because ε-SVR and ν-SVR are kernel methods that are more common than RVR, it is desirable to investigate the differences between the performances of all three methods. Furthermore, dimensionality reduction via PCA may also influence the accuracy of age estimation.

As summarized in Table 2.4, age estimation tended to be more accurate when the dimensionality of the data was reduced to 410 principal compo-

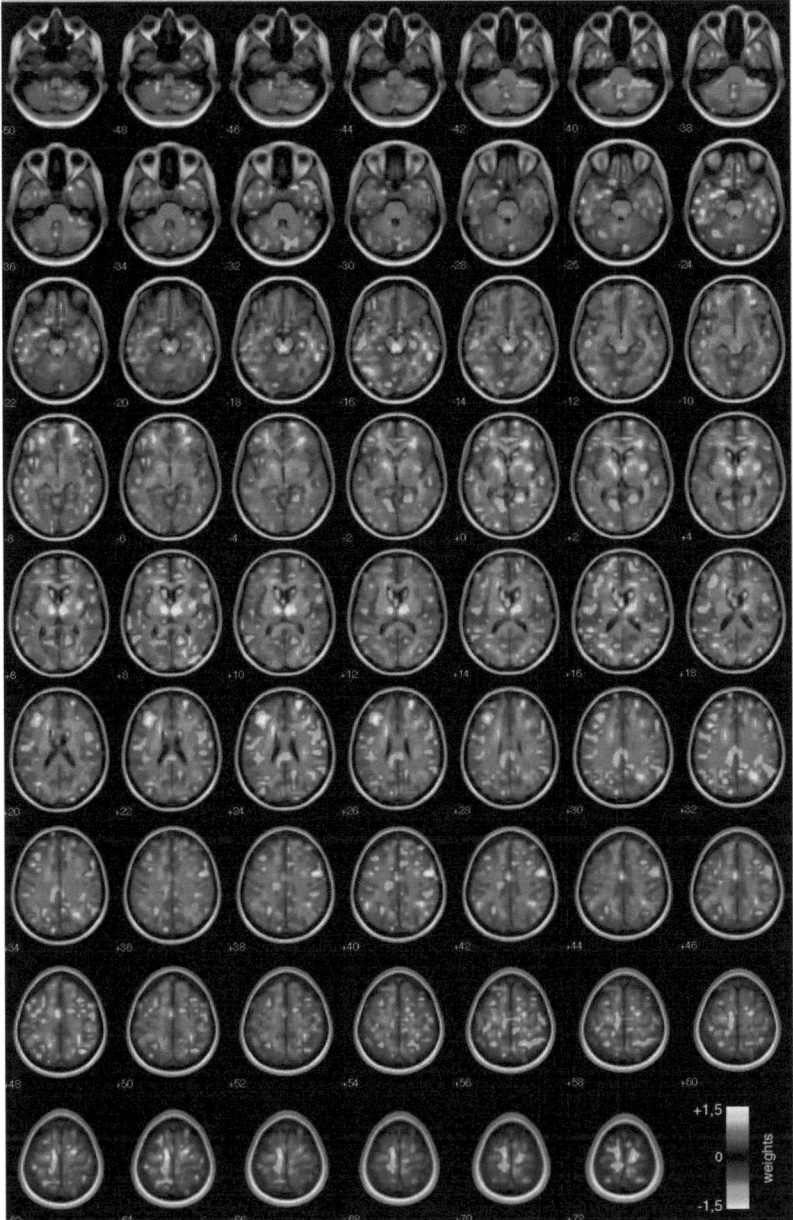

Figure 2.5: To illustrate the most important features that were used by the RVR for estimating the age based on MRI data, weights below the 5th and above the 95th quartile are displayed, overlaid on the normalized mean image of TRAIN1–3. Color scale indicates the weight (i.e., the importance of the voxel location for regression). [Figure and legend from Franke et al. 2010.]

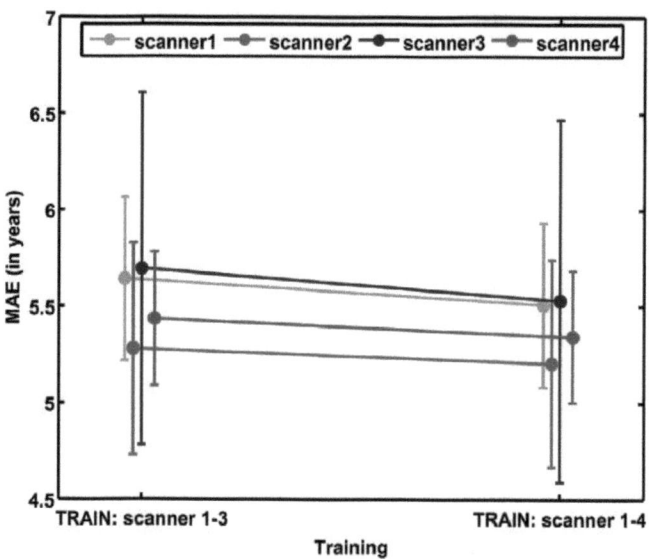

Figure 2.6: To test for the effect of scanners on prediction accuracy, the IXI data set (scanners 1–3) as well as sample TEST4 (scanner 4) were randomly split into four groups. The first training run included 75% of the IXI data. For the modified training run, 75% of the TEST4 sample was added to the IXI training set. Age estimation was performed on the remaining data. Results were averaged over 20 trials and are shown for each scanner separately. Error bars depict the standard error of the mean (SEM). [Figure and legend modified from Franke et al. 2010.]

nents and RVR was used for model calculation (also see Figure 2.7). On the other hand, especially when using principal components, the performance of ε-SVR and ν-SVR was not stable but depended heavily on the choice of its parameters. While using sample-dependent parameters as proposed in Cherkassky and Ma (2004) and Chalimourda et al. (2004), the MAEs reached up to 5 years and thus were comparable to the MAE from the RVR model. Without using sample-dependent parameters or performing a grid search to find optimal parameters for ε-SVR and ν-SVR, but instead using the default values (i.e., $C = 1$; $\varepsilon = 0.1$ and $\nu = 0.5$, respectively), the MAE for estimating the age with reduced data was substantially worse – scoring 8 and 9 years, respectively (Figure 2.7).

Table 2.4: Results of training and testing the age estimation model utilizing different regression methods, each with and without dimension reduction via PCA. MAE (in years) is shown, with the best results in **bold**.

		TEST1–3	TEST4	TEST1–3 + TEST4
RVR	PCA	**4.61**	5.44	**4.98**
	noPCA	4.96	5.57	5.23
ε-SVR	PCA	4.85	5.42	5.10
(C = 98; ε = 0.064)	noPCA	4.85	5.51	5.14
ν-SVR	PCA	4.85	5.51	5.14
(C = 20500; ν = 0.54)	noPCA	4.85	5.51	5.14
ε-SVR	PCA	9.82	5.97	8.12
(C = 1; ε = 0.1)	noPCA	4.76	5.39	5.04
ν-SVR	PCA	11.06	6.38	9.00
(C = 1; ν = 0.5)	noPCA	4.72	**5.36**	5.00

Taking a closer look at the number of principal components used in training and testing the age estimation model (using RVR), the accuracy continuously improved with an increasing number of principal components, with a convergence to the smallest MAE at about the first 350 principal components (Figure 2.8). Severe overfitting was prevented due to the inherent characteristics of RVM.

Furthermore, training and testing the age estimation model utilizing RVR or SVR was computationally fast, with a processing time for training and testing the reduced data of only a few seconds on MAC OS X, Version 10.4.11, Dual 2.5 GHz PowerPC G5 (Figure 2.9).

2.4.4 Comparison of variations in data preprocessing (affine vs. modulated, smoothing, and spatial resolution)

With respect to preprocessing of the MRI data, we compared different kinds of registration (AF versus NL), different sizes of the smoothing kernel (S4 versus S8), and different spatial resolutions (R3, R4, and R8). The MAE of

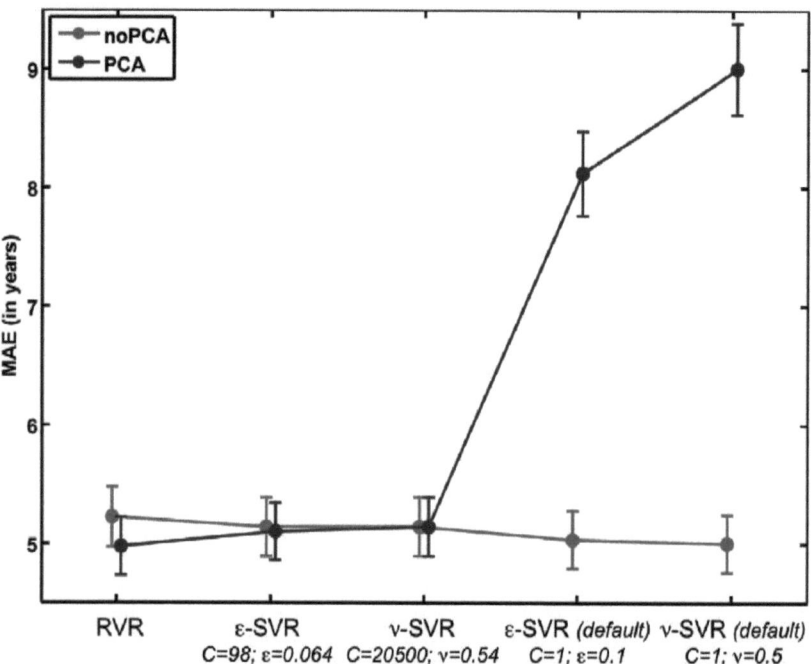

Figure 2.7: Age estimation tended to be best when the dimensionality of the data was reduced via PCA (dark blue) and RVR was used for model calculation. With the reduced data, the performance of ε-SVR and ν-SVR was not stable but depended heavily on the choice of parameters. Error bars depict the SEM. [Figure and legend modified from Franke et al. 2010.]

the age estimations ranged from 4.98 to 5.45 years, and the most accurate predictions occurred with affine registration and a smoothing kernel of 8 mm. The influence of spatial resolution was negligible (Table 2.5, Figure 2.10).

2.4.5 Influence of the size of training data

Figure 2.11 illustrates that the size of the training data set had a strong effect on the accuracy of age estimation. Whereas the full data set (n = 410 subjects) produced an MAE of less than 5 years, using only one half (n = 205) or a quarter (n = 103) of the training data set for training the age estimation model produced MAEs of 5.2 and 5.6 years, respectively.

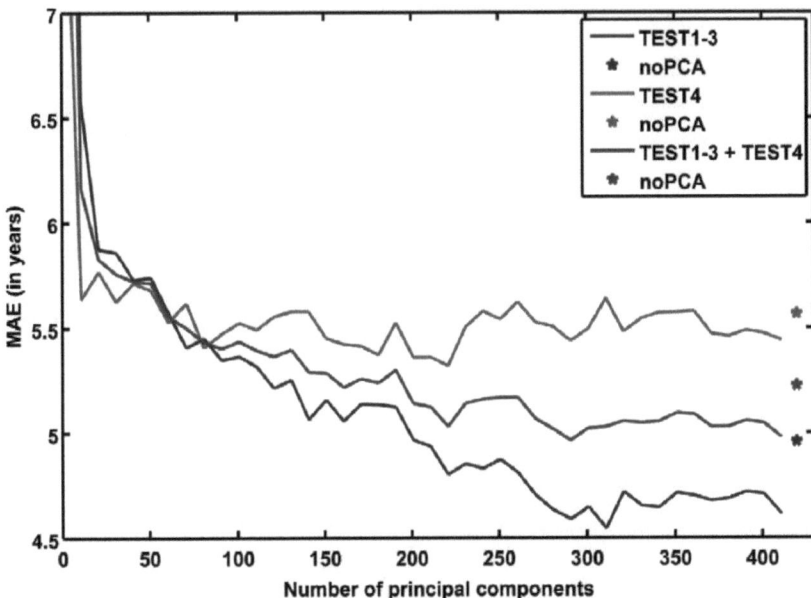

Figure 2.8: The accuracy of the age estimation model (using RVR) continuously improves with an increasing number of principal components, observing a convergence to the smallest MAE at about the first 350 principal components. MAEs shown for each test sample separately as well as for both test samples together (purple). Star symbols represent MAEs resulting from training the age estimation model without data reduction, but utilizing the preprocessed MRI data. [Figure and legend modified from Franke et al. 2010.]

2.4.6 Comparing the influence of the various parameters

Merging the set of all adjustable parameters and methodologies, it can be seen in Figure 2.12 that the accuracy of age estimation depended mostly on the number of subjects used for training. The method for preprocessing the T1-weighted MRI images also showed a strong influence on the accuracy of age estimation, again favoring affine registration with a broad smoothing kernel. Furthermore, reducing the dimensionality of data via PCA also had a moderate effect on the MAE.

Table 2.5: Results of analyses with respect to registration method [affine (AF) vs. non-linear (NL)], size of the smoothing kernel [4 mm (S4) vs. 8 mm (S8)], and spatial resolution [3 mm (R3), 4 mm (R4), 8 mm (R8)]. Results are shown in terms of MAE (in years). The best results are marked in **bold**.

Registration	NL			AF					
Smoothing kernel	S4			S4			S8		
Spatial resolution	R3	R4	R8	R3	R4	R8	R3	R4	R8
TEST1–3	5.02	5.05	5.28	5.21	5.18	5.19	4.67	4.72	**4.61**
TEST4	4.98	**4.96**	5.19	5.30	5.38	5.77	5.49	5.54	5.44
TEST1–3 + TEST4	5.00	5.01	5.24	5.25	5.27	5.45	5.03	5.08	**4.98**

2.4.7 Estimating the age of patients with early AD

The age estimation framework was applied to T1-weighted MRI images of the NO group and the AD group sampled from the ADNI database. The *Brain-AGE* score was calculated for each subject. For the AD group, the mean *BrainAGE* score was 10 years, implying a systematically higher estimated than true age based on the MRI data (Figure 2.13). This deviation was highly significant ($p < 0.001$, $df = 332$).

2.5 Discussion

For estimating the age of healthy subjects from T1-weighted MRI scans, we propose a framework that includes automatic preprocessing of the images, dimension reduction via PCA, training of an RVM for regression with a polynomial kernel of degree 1, and finally estimating the age of the subjects from the two test samples TEST1–3 and TEST4. This age estimating framework turns out to be a straightforward method to accurately and reliably estimate age with as little preprocessing and parameter optimization as possible. The additional challenge consisted of combining images from three different scanners for training and testing with an additional testing set from a fourth scanner not included during the training step.

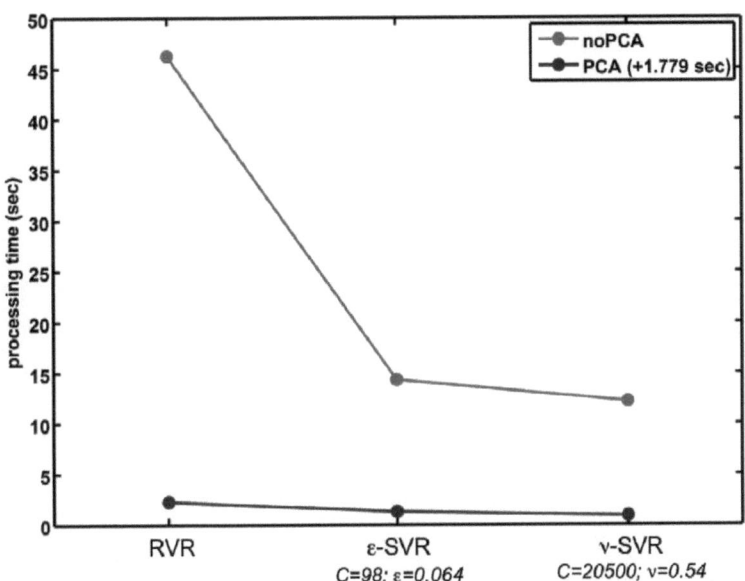

Figure 2.9: Training and testing the age estimation model utilizing RVR or SVR needed only a few seconds on MAC OS X, Version 10.4.11, Dual 2.5 GHz PowerPC G5 if the dimensions were reduced to 410 principal components (dark blue). [Figure and legend modified from Franke et al. 2010.]

Using MRI data from more than 650 healthy subjects aged between 19 – 86 and scanned on different scanners, the age estimation with RVR showed excellent performance for both test samples, with an overall MAE of only 5 years and a correlation of $r = 0.92$ between the estimated and the real age. Although the data in TEST4 were collected on a scanner that was not included in the training step, the performance measures for age estimation showed only minor differences to those of TEST1–3. We did not detect any systematical bias in the age estimation with older age or gender.

Including data from the fourth "unknown" scanner into the training sample did not improve the overall accuracy of age prediction. This could be due to the age range of the samples. TEST4 comprised data from subjects aged between 20 – 59 years, which were already frequently represented in the original training sample TRAIN1–3. On the other hand, adding data from healthy

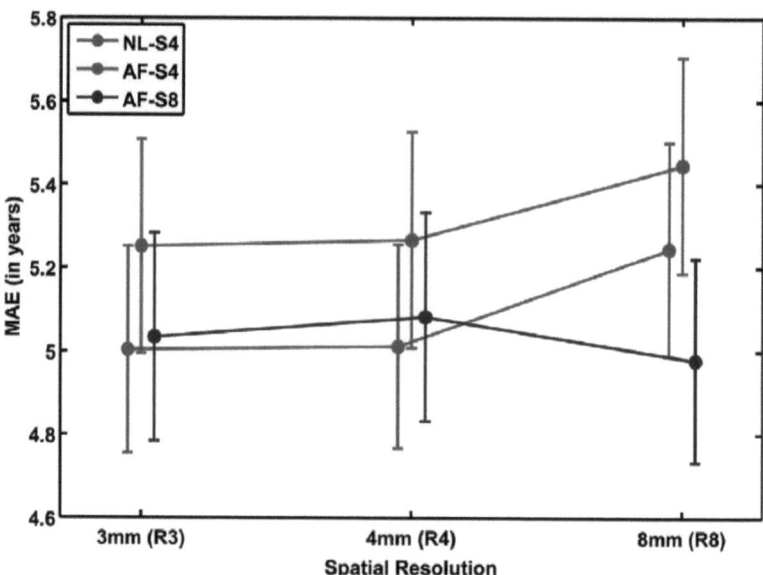

Figure 2.10: Comparing the different kinds of registration [affine (AF) vs. non-linear (NL)], different sizes of the smoothing kernel [4 mm (S4) vs. 8 mm (S8)], and different spatial resolutions [3 mm (R3), 4 mm (R4), 8 mm (R8)], the MAE of age estimation changes only slightly, with the most accurate age estimation obtained for affine registration and a smoothing kernel of 8 mm (dark blue). Error bars depict the SEM. [Figure and legend modified from Franke et al. 2010.]

subjects with an age range of 60 – 90 would probably have had a stronger influence on the performance of RVR. Thus, with respect to combining data from different scanners, our results are in line with those of Klöppel et al. (2008b). They indicate that the effect of scanner is sufficiently different from that of the aging process that they could be separated by the regression method. These encouraging results suggest this framework as an accurate, scanner-independent, and efficient method for age estimation in healthy subjects.

In RVR, the type of kernel is the only parameter that has to be defined by the user. In contrast, in ε-SVR and ν-SVR, another two parameters have to be chosen and can decrease the performance if they are not optimized for the specific sample. Age estimation with RVR tends to be slightly better with

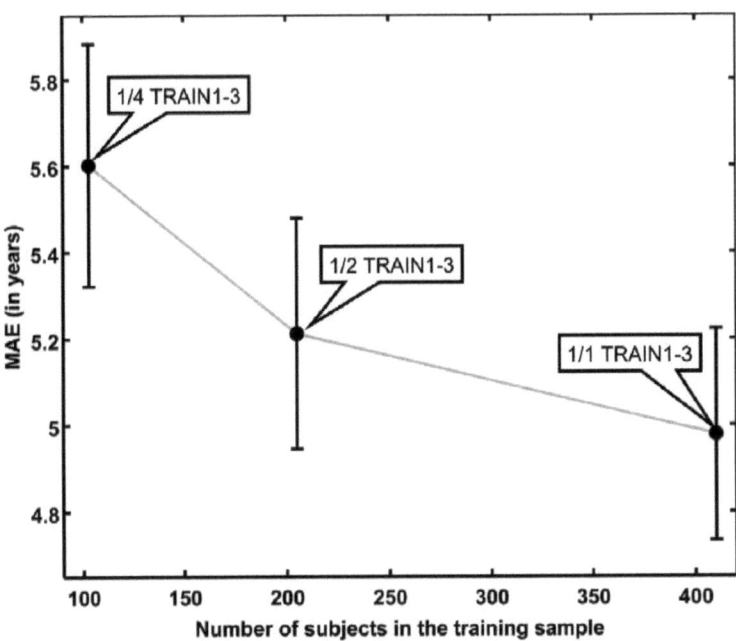

Figure 2.11: Shown is the influence of the size of trainings data set. Whereas the full data (1/1 TRAIN1–3) set produced an MAE of less than 5 years, taking only one half (1/2 TRAIN1–3) or a quarter (1/4 TRAIN1–3) of the training data set for computing the age estimation model produced MAEs of 5.2 and 5.6 years, respectively. Error bars depict the SEM. [Figure and legend modified from Franke et al. 2010.]

PCA than without. Furthermore, using the principal components for training and testing with RVR only needed a few seconds and thus is significantly faster than using the full original data set (Figure 2.9).

We decided to use PCA for data reduction because of several reasons: it is a rather simple and commonly used method, and a number of fast implementations exist that are compatible with large data sets. Furthermore, when testing other data reduction or feature selection methods (e.g., Recursive Feature Elimination; Guyon et al., 2002; Guyon and Elisseeff, 2003), we did not observe any improvement in accuracy of age estimation. Also, van der Maaten (2007) reported that the results of their experiments on artificial and

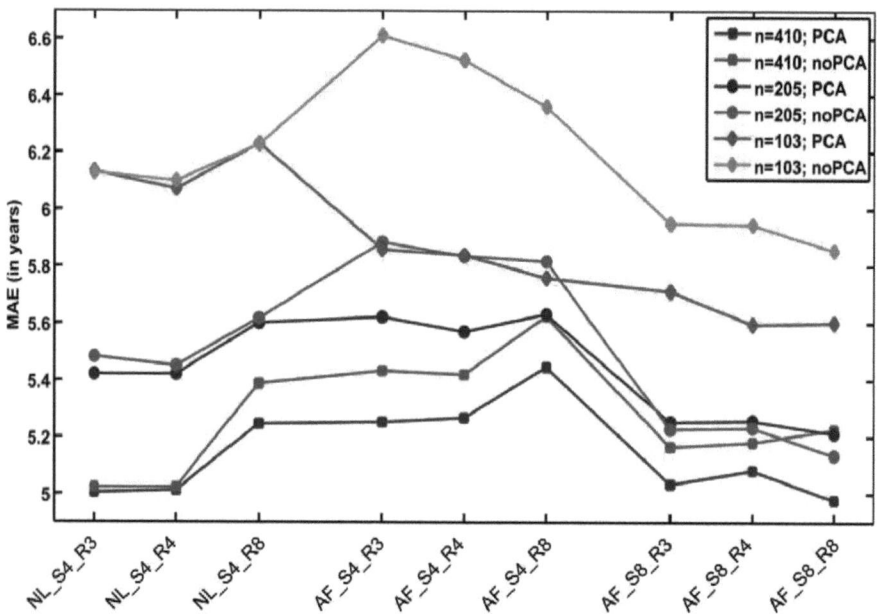

Figure 2.12: Integrating the influences of the various parameters: the accuracy of age estimation es- sentially depends on the number of subjects used for training the age estimation model (blue lines: full training set TRAIN1–3); the method for preprocessing the T1-weighted MRI images also showed a strong influence on the accuracy of age estimation; and data reduction via PCA only had a moderate effect on the MAE. [Figure and legend modified from Franke et al. 2010.]

natural data sets indicate no clear improvement of non-linear techniques (for example, Isomap or Laplacian Eigenmaps and others) over traditional PCA.

The number of training samples was found to have the strongest influence on the accuracy of age prediction. Our results suggest that the preprocessing of the T1-weighted MRI images can be done fairly rapidly by performing an affine registration only with a large smoothing kernel (e.g., 8 mm). Furthermore, given limited computing time and memory, a coarse spatial resolution (e.g., 8 mm) can be used without losing estimation accuracy. A dimensionality reduction of the data can be conducted using PCA, which tends to improve the accuracy and at the same time speeds up the computing of the RVR model and estimating the age values of the test subjects.

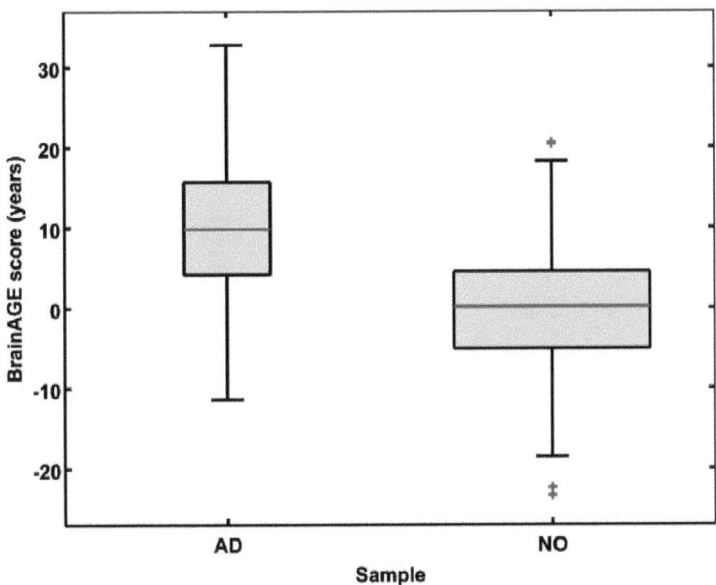

Figure 2.13: Shown are box plots with *BrainAGE* scores (in years) for the two samples from the ADNI database (AD with CDR = 1, NO with CDR = 0). The gray boxes contain the values between the 25th and 75th percentiles of the samples, including the median (red line). Lines extending above and below each box symbolize data within 1.5 times the interquartile range (outliers are displayed with a red +). The width of the boxes depends on the sample size. [Figure and legend modified from Franke et al. 2010.]

Finally, our age estimation framework has the potential to provide clinically relevant information. With a mean *BrainAGE* score of +10 years, the subjects with early AD showed signs of accelerated brain aging.

In conclusion, our age estimation framework could potentially help to recognize or indicate faster brain atrophy before the onset of clinical symptoms, thus contributing to an early diagnosis of neurodegenerative diseases and facilitate early treatment or a preventative intervention. Depending on the availability of subject data, future explorations could include applying this framework to other neurodegenerative diseases, evaluating the therapeutic effect of drugs or other treatment modalities, and to predict either the severity of symptoms or the possible rate of cognitive decline.[6]

---

[6] **Acknowledgments:** The clinical data used in the preparation of this article were obtained from the Alzheimer's Disease Neuroimaging Initiative (ADNI) database (www.loni.ucla.edu/ADNI). The ADNI was launched in 2003 by the National Institute on Aging (NIA), the National Institute of Biomedical Imaging and Bioengineering (NIBIB), the Food and Drug Administration (FDA), private pharmaceutical companies and non-profit organizations, as a $60 million, 5-year public-private partnership. The Foundation for the National Institutes of Health (www.fnih.org) coordinates the private sector participation of the $60 million ADNI public-private partnership that was begun by the National Institute on Aging (NIA) and supported by the National Institutes of Health. To date, more than $27 million has been provided to the Foundation for NIH by Abbott, AstraZeneca AB, Bayer Schering Pharma AG, Bristol-Myers Squibb, Eisai Global Clinical Development, Elan Corporation, Genentech, GE Healthcare, GlaxoSmithKline, Innogenetics, Johnson and Johnson, Eli Lilly and Co., Merck and Co., Inc., Novartis AG, Pfizer Inc., F. Hoffmann-La Roche, Schering-Plough, Synarc Inc., and Wyeth as well as non-profit partners, the Alzheimer's Association and the Institute for the Study of Aging.

Chapter 3.

Longitudinal changes in individual *BrainAGE* in healthy aging, mild cognitive impairment, and Alzheimer's disease [7]

3.1 Abstract

We recently proposed a novel method that aggregates the multidimensional aging pattern across the brain to a single value. This method proved to provide stable and reliable estimates of brain aging – even across different scanners. While investigating longitudinal changes in *BrainAGE* in about 400 elderly subjects, we discovered that patients with Alzheimer's disease (AD) and subjects who had converted to AD within 3 years showed accelerated brain atrophy by +6 years at baseline. An additional increase in *BrainAGE* accumulated to a score of about +9 years during follow-up. Accelerated brain aging was related to prospective cognitive decline and disease severity. In conclusion, the *BrainAGE* framework indicates discrepancies in brain aging and could thus serve as an indicator for cognitive functioning in the future.

3.2 Introduction

During normal brain development and aging, the brain is affected by progressive (e.g., cell growth and myelination) and by regressive (e.g., cell death and atrophy) neuronal processes (Silk and Wood, 2011). Those processes have been found to follow a specific pattern, with gray matter (GM) volume increasing in the first years of life and thereafter decreasing continuously; and with white matter (WM) volume increasing steadily until around the age of 20 when it plateaus (Good et al., 2001; Pfefferbaum et al., 1994). Healthy brain aging has been found to follow a specific heterogeneous and complex pattern

---

[7] Research article [published as: Franke, K., Gaser, C., and Alzheimer's Disease Neuroimaging Initiative (2012). Longitudinal changes in individual *BrainAGE* in healthy aging, mild cognitive impairment, and Alzheimer's disease. *GeroPsych*, 25(4):235–245.]

of atrophy across the adult lifespan (Good et al., 2001), with normal age-related GM decline being inversely related to the phylogenetic origin of each respective region, i.e., younger structures being the last to mature as well as being more vulnerable to neurodegeneration (Terribilli et al., 2011; Toga et al., 2006).

With the growing number of studies that have investigated both normal and abnormal age-related brain changes, most major neuropsychiatric disorders are now thought to arise due to deviations from normal brain development (Gogtay and Thompson, 2010). Also diseases such as Alzheimer's disease (AD) and schizophrenia alter brain structures in diverse and abnormal modes (Ashburner et al., 2003; Meda et al., 2008). AD in particular is widely assumed to reflect accelerated aging (Cao et al., 2010; Jones et al., 2011; Saetre et al., 2011), with accelerated age-related changes in brain atrophy being already evident at the stage of mild cognitive impairment (MCI), i.e., the prodromal stage of AD (Driscoll et al., 2009; Spulber et al., 2010). Additional evidence for this view was recently provided by showing that the atrophied regions detected in AD patients are largely overlapping with regions showing a normal age-related decline in age-matched healthy control subjects (Dukart et al., 2011).

Given the widespread but well-ordered brain tissue loss that occurs as a function of age-based processes, a straight-forward and efficient solution might be to model healthy brain aging in order to subsequently identify abnormal aging processes and accelerated brain atrophy before the onset of upcoming clinical symptoms. Recently, we introduced a new approach based on structural magnet resonance imaging (MRI) data that enables to reliably estimate the brain age of any given subject (Franke et al., 2010). By employing kernel regression methods in a large training database, the complex, multidimensional aging patterns across the whole brain are detected and finally aggregated to a single value, i.e., the estimated brain age (Figure 1.4A; page

21). The individual discrepancies between estimated and chronological age were termed *"Brain Age Gap Estimation"* (*BrainAGE*) score, with observed differences in *BrainAGE* scores being interpreted as originating from structural brain changes that show the pattern of accelerated (or decelerated) aging. Consequently, although only one MRI scan per subject is employed, the degree of acceleration or deceleration of brain aging can be quantified directly in terms of years, allowing a wide range of analyses and predictions on an individual level. For example, if a 70-year-old individual has a deviating *BrainAGE* score of +5 years, this means that this individual shows the typical atrophy pattern of a 75-year-old individual (Figure 1.4B; page 21). The framework comprises well-established and fully automatic processing steps of the MRI data, combines data from different scanners, and accurately estimates the age of healthy individuals with a correlation of $r = 0.92$ between estimated and chronological age. Furthermore, this brain-age estimation model has showed its potential to provide clinically relevant information by reporting a statistically significant, positive deviation of 10 years between estimated and chronological age in AD patients from the Alzheimer's Disease Neuroimaging Initiative (ADNI) database, indicating structural brain changes that show the pattern of accelerated aging (Franke et al., 2010). Additionally, a slightly modified *BrainAGE* approach recently provided a reliable reference curve based on structural MRI data, allowing for the prediction of structural brain maturation and a fast identification of developmental delays in childhood and adolescence (Franke et al., 2012b).

By implementing this new method of brain-age estimation, our present studies further analyze the stability and reliability of the *BrainAGE* approach, utilizing two subsamples that have (1) a short delay between two scans of the same subject on the same scanner (1.5T) as well as (2) two scans of the same subjects with two different field strengths (1.5T and 3.0T). Second, within a follow-up period of up to 4 years we explored the patterns of longitudinal changes in individual *BrainAGE* and quantified about 400 cognitively normal, MCI, and AD subjects. Further, we related discrepancies in brain aging to prospective cognitive functioning and disease severity.

3.3 Methods
3.3.1 ADNI database

Part of the data used in the preparation of this article were obtained from the ADNI database[8]. The ADNI was launched in 2003 by the National Institute on Aging (NIA), the National Institute of Biomedical Imaging and Bioengineering (NIBIB), the Food and Drug Administration (FDA), private pharmaceutical companies, and non-profit organizations, as a $60 million, 5-year public-private partnership. The primary goal of ADNI was to test whether serial MRI, positron emission tomography (PET), other biological markers as well as clinical and neuropsychological assessment can be combined to measure the progression of MCI and early AD. Determination of sensitive and specific markers of very early AD progression should aid researchers and clinicians in developing new treatments and monitoring their effectiveness as well as lessening the time and cost of clinical trials.

The principal investigator of this initiative is Michael W. Weiner, MD, VA Medical Center and University of California, San Francisco. ADNI is the result of efforts of many coinvestigators from a broad range of academic institutions and private corporations, and subjects have been recruited from over 50 sites across the United States and Canada. The initial goal of ADNI was to recruit 800 adults, aged 55 – 90, to participate in the research; approximately 200 cognitively normal older individuals to be followed for 3 years; 400 people with MCI to be followed for 3 years; and 200 people with early AD to be followed for 2 years. For up-to-date information, see www.adni-info.org.

---

[8] http://adni.loni.ucla.edu

3.3.2 Subjects

To train the age estimation framework, we used T1-weighted MRI data of 560 healthy subjects (249 males) from the publicly accessible IXI cohort[9] (data downloaded in September 2011) aged 20 – 86 years, which were collected on three different scanners (Philips 1.5T, General Electric 1.5T, Philips 3.0T).

Before analyzing the individual patterns of longitudinal *BrainAGE* changes, the stability of *BrainAGE* estimations within the same subjects were explored using two different subsamples. The first test sample included structural MRI data of 20 healthy subjects (aged 19 – 34 years) from the Open Access Series of Imaging Studies database (OASIS[10]; Marcus et al., 2007), for whom a short-delay (less than 90 days) double scan on the same scanner was available (Siemens 1.5T). The second test sample included 1.5T as well as 3.0T structural MRI data (acquired within a short delay) of 60 healthy non-demented elderly subjects (aged 60 – 87 years) from the ADNI database (data downloaded in May 2010). The characteristics of all three samples are given in Table 3.1.

To investigate the longitudinal pattern of *BrainAGE* changes in healthy aging, MCI, and AD, a third test sample included all subjects from the ADNI database for whom at least the baseline scan and one follow-up scan were

Table 3.1: Characteristics of the subjects in the training group (IXI) and both test samples (OASIS and ADNI) double-scanned within a short delay (< 90 days).

	Training sample	Test samples	
	IXI	OASIS	ADNI
No. subjects	560	20	60
Males / Females	249 / 311	8 / 12	22 / 38
Age mean (SD)	48.6 (16.5)	23.4 (4.0)	75.2 (4.8)
Age range	20 – 86	19 – 34	60 – 87
No. of MRI scanners (1.5T / 3.0T)	2 / 1	1 / 0	26 / 26

---

[9] www.brain-development.org
[10] www.oasis-brains.org

available (1.5T). Adopting the diagnostic classification at baseline and follow-up, subjects were grouped as (i) *NO* (healthy subjects) if diagnosis was NO at baseline and 3-year follow-up (n = 108); (ii) *sMCI* (stable MCI) if diagnosis was MCI at baseline and 3-year follow-up (n = 36); (iii) *pMCI* (progressive MCI) if diagnosis was MCI at baseline and AD at some follow-up, without reversion to MCI or NO (n = 112); (iv) *AD* patients if diagnosis was AD at baseline, without reversion (n = 150). For further analyses we used baseline and follow-up test scores of the cognitive scales: Alzheimer's Disease Assessment Scale (ADAS; range 0 – 85, with higher test scores being related to worse cognitive functioning; Mohs and Cohen, 1988; Mohs, 1996), global Clinical Dementia Rating Scale (CDR; range 0 – 3, with 0 denoting cognitively healthy, 0.5 denoting mild cognitive impairments, and a score of 1 or above denoting AD; Morris, 1993), and Mini-Mental State Examination (MMSE; range 0 – 30, with lower scores being related to higher disease severity; Cockrell and Folstein, 1988). The baseline and follow-up characteristics of this test sample are given in Table 3.2.

Table 3.2: Characteristics of the ADNI test sample for longitudinal analyses.

		NO	sMCI	pMCI	AD
	No. subjects	108	36	112	150
	Males / Females	61 / 47	30 / 6	67 / 45	76 / 74
Baseline	Age mean (SD)	75.6 (5.0)	77.0 (6.1)	74.5 (7.4)	74.6 (7.6)
	MMSE mean (SD)	29.2 (0.9)	27.4 (1.9)	26.6 (1.7)	23.4 (1.9)
	CDR mean (SD)	0.00 (0.00)	0.50 (0.00)	0.50 (0.00)	0.73 (0.25)
	ADAS mean (SD)	8.8 (3.8)	17.3 (5.9)	21.8 (5.7)	28.8 (7.8)
	No. scans (SD)	5.0 (0.8)	5.9 (0.9)	5.2 (1.4)	3.4 (0.7)
Follow-up	Follow-up duration in days (SD)	1194 (261)	1114 (244)	969 (360)	609 (222)
	Age at last scan (SD)	78.9 (5.0)	80.1 (6.0)	77.2 (7.6)	76.3 (7.7)
	MMSE mean (SD)	29.0 (1.3)	27.1 (2.6)	21.6 (4.3)	19.3 (5.6)
	CDR mean (SD)	0.06 (0.16)	0.49 (0.15)	0.92 (0.42)	1.27 (0.67)
	ADAS mean (SD)	10.1 (5.4)	17.6 (6.5)	32.5 (9.5)	38.1 (12.1)

3.3.3 Preprocessing of MRI data and data reduction

Preprocessing of the T1-weighted images was done using the SPM8 package[11] and the VBM8 toolbox[12], running under MATLAB. All T1-weighted images were corrected for bias-field inhomogeneities, then spatially normalized and segmented into GM, WM, and cerebrospinal fluid (CSF) within the same generative model (Ashburner and Friston, 2005). The segmentation procedure was further extended by accounting for partial volume effects (Tohka et al., 2004), by applying adaptive maximum a posteriori estimations (Rajapakse et al., 1997), and by using a hidden Markov random field model (Cuadra et al., 2005) as described previously (Gaser, 2009). The images were processed with affine registration and smoothed with 4 mm full-width-at-half-maximum (FWHM) smoothing kernels.

3.3.4 *BrainAGE* framework

The *BrainAGE* framework utilizes a high-dimensional pattern recognition method, i.e., relevance vector regression (RVR; Tipping, 2001), to model healthy brain aging. RVR was introduced by Tipping (2000) as a Bayesian alternative to support vector machines (SVM), but is easier to use since all model parameters are automatically estimated by the learning procedure itself. More details can be found in Bishop (2006), Schölkopf and Smola (2002), and Tipping (2000). Recently, the *BrainAGE* framework proved to be a reliable, scanner-independent, and efficient method for age estimation in healthy subjects (Franke et al., 2010). It resulted in a correlation of $r = 0.92$ between the estimated and the real age in the test samples, and a mean absolute error (MAE) of 5 years. Furthermore, the study identified the number of training samples as the critical factor for prediction accuracy.

---

[11] www.fil.ion.ucl.ac.uk/spm
[12] http://dbm.neuro.uni-jena.de

In general, the age regression model is trained with the chronological age and preprocessed whole brain structural MRI data of the training sample, resulting in a complex model of healthy brain aging (Figure 1.4A, left; page 21). Subsequently, the brain age of a test subject can be estimated using the individual tissue-classified MRI data, aggregating the complex, multidimensional aging pattern across the whole brain into one single value (Figure 1.4A, right; page 21). The difference between estimated and chronological age results in the *BrainAGE* score, which consequently directly quantifies the amount of acceleration or deceleration in brain aging (Figure 1.4B; page 21). For training the model as well as for predicting individual brain ages, we used "The Spider"[13], a freely available toolbox running under MATLAB. For more detailed information please refer to Franke et al. (2010).

Within this study, the linear combination of whole brain GM and WM images were used to train the *BrainAGE* framework. Data reduction was performed by applying principal component analysis (PCA), utilizing the "MATLAB Toolbox for Dimensionality Reduction"[14]. PCA was performed only on the training sample. The estimated transformation parameters were subsequently applied to the test samples, allowing estimation of individual brain ages based on baseline MRI data. The difference between the estimated and the chronological age resulted in the *BrainAGE* score, indicating accelerated (positive values) or decelerated (negative values) brain aging.

3.3.5 Statistical analysis

In the first analysis, the intraclass correlation coeffcient (ICC; two-way random single measures) as well as Student's t-test was calculated for each test sample separately to assess the conformity and stability of *BrainAGE* estima-

---
[13] www.kyb.mpg.de/bs/people/spider/main.html
[14] http://ict.ewi.tudelft.nl/~lvandermaaten/Home.html

tions across several MRI scans within a short delay (OASIS) and across different scanner field-strengths (ADNI).

In the second analysis, the longitudinal changes in individual *BrainAGE* scores, which were corrected for age and gender, were fitted against days from baseline with a multivariate linear regression model. Baseline *BrainAGE* scores, *BrainAGE* scores at last visit, and longitudinal changes in *BrainAGE* were compared among the four diagnostic groups using an analysis of variance (ANOVA). Post-hoc analyses (with Bonferroni adjustment to compensate for multiple comparisons) were conducted to further explore significant group differences. The relationship between *BrainAGE* scores and cognitive scales (i.e., MMSE, CDR, ADAS) were explored using Pearson's linear correlation coeffcients. ICC was calculated using SPSS. All other statistical testing was performed using MATLAB.

3.4 Results
3.4.1 Stability of *BrainAGE* estimations

The *BrainAGE* estimations within the same subjects proved to be stable across a short delay between two scans as well as across scanners. In the OASIS subsample, in which the subjects had a short delay between two scans on the same scanner (1.5T), the brain-age estimations resulted in mean (SD) raw *BrainAGE* scores of 13.8 (6.1) years for the 1st and 12.8 (5.6) years for the 2nd scan (Figure 3.1, left). The raw *BrainAGE* scores derived from the 1st as well as 2nd scan significantly differed from a zero mean ($p < 0.001$), but not among each other ($p = 0.60$). The correlation between the raw *BrainAGE* scores derived from the 1st and 2nd scan data resulted in $r = 0.93$ ($p < 0.001$). Thus, the results suggest a systematical data-specific offset at each of both scanning time points. For illustration reasons and / or better interpretability of the results, this offset can be easily adjusted by a linear shift, i.e., setting the *BrainAGE* scores to a zero group mean (Figure 3.1,

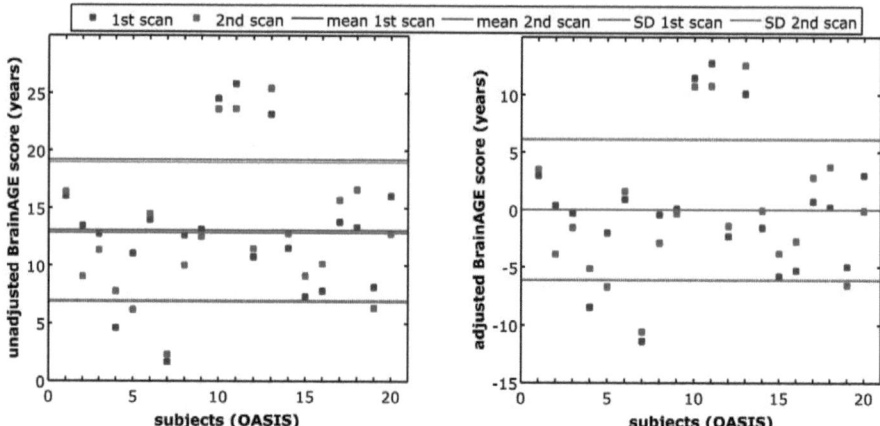

Figure 3.1: Unadjusted *(left panel)* and offset-adjusted *(right panel)* BrainAGE scores for double-scanned OASIS subjects on the same scanner within a short delay. ICC between the *BrainAGE* scores calculated from the 1st and 2nd scan was 0.93. [Figure and legend from Franke et al. 2012a.]

right). Linearly adjusting for the offset at each scanning time point separately, resulted in a correlation between raw and adjusted *BrainAGE* scores of $r = 0.996$ ($p < 0.001$). The ICC between the *BrainAGE* scores calculated from the 1st and 2nd scan was 0.93 [95% confidence interval (CI): 0.83 – 0.97], demonstrating strong stability of the estimated *BrainAGE* scores across several MRI scans.

The ADNI subsample, which included only non-demented subjects who had two baseline scans from MRI scanners of two different field strengths (1.5T and 3.0T) showed mean (SD) raw *BrainAGE* scores of –5.9 (7.0) years for the 1.5T data and –9.1 (6.6) years for the 3.0T data (Figure 3.2, left), with a correlation between both scans of $r = 0.91$ ($p < 0.001$). The raw *BrainAGE* scores derived from the 1.5T as well as 3.0T data significantly differed from a zero mean ($p < 0.001$). These results additionally suggest a strong dependency of brain-age estimation on field strength, with 1.5T MRI data resulting in larger *BrainAGE* scores than those derived with 3.0T MRI data. Again, this offset can be easily adjusted by a linear shift as described above (Figure 3.1,

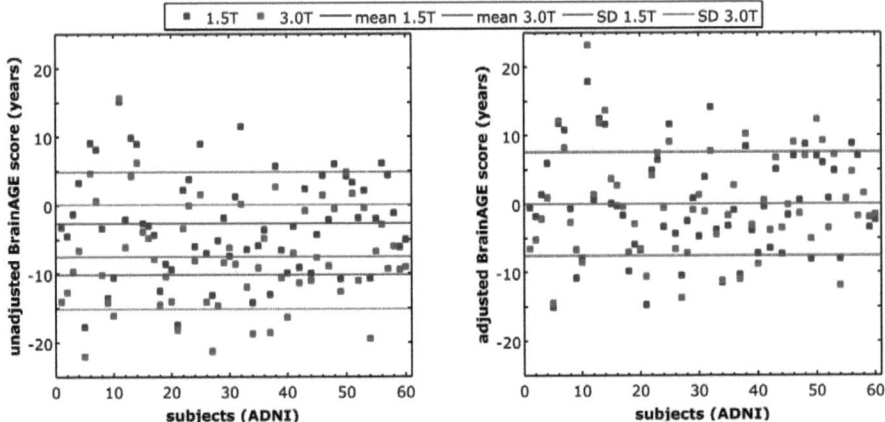

Figure 3.2: Unadjusted *(left panel)* and offset-adjusted *(right panel) BrainAGE* scores for double-scanned ADNI subjects on 1.5T and 3.0T scanner within a short delay. ICC between the *BrainAGE* scores calculated from the 1.5T and 3.0T scan was 0.90. [Figure and legend from Franke et al. 2012a.]

right). After linearly adjusting for the field strength-specific offset, Student's t-test resulted in no difference between the *BrainAGE* scores calculated from the 1.5T and 3.0T scan (p = 1.00). ICC between the *BrainAGE* scores calculated from the 1.5T and 3.0T scan was 0.90 [CI: 0.84 – 0.94], demonstrating strong stability of the estimated *BrainAGE* scores across different field strengths. Taken together, these results suggest that the *BrainAGE* framework reliably estimates individual brain age based on structural MRI data.

3.4.2 Longitudinal *BrainAGE* estimation

In the longitudinal ADNI sample, the baseline *BrainAGE* scores differed among the four groups (F = 26.8, p < 0.001). For better interpretability, all individual *BrainAGE* scores were adjusted by a linear shift determined in the NO group (as described in section 3.4.1). Thus, the baseline *BrainAGE* scores resulted in the following group means: NO = –0.30 years, sMCI = –0.48 years, pMCI = 6.19 years, and AD = 6.67 years (Figure 3.3A). Post-hoc t-tests showed significant differences between NO/sMCI vs. pMCI/AD

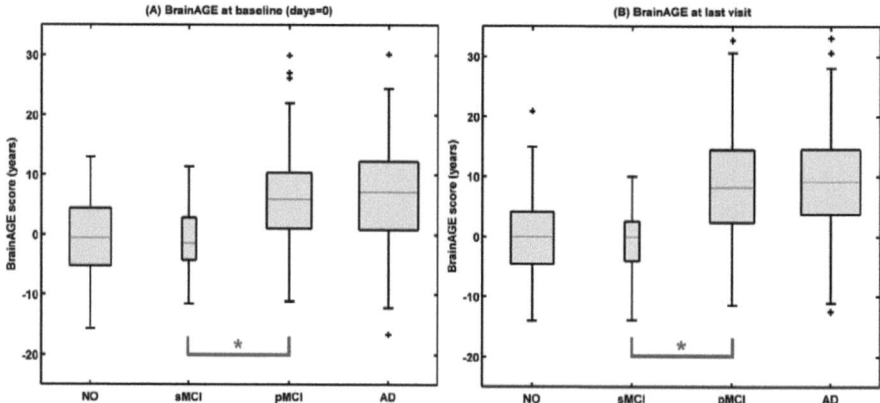

Figure 3.3: Box plots of **(A)** baseline *BrainAGE* scores and **(B)** *BrainAGE* scores of last MRI scans for all diagnostic groups. Post-hoc t-tests showed significant differences between NO/sMCI vs. pMCI/AD ($p < 0.05$) at both time measurements. The gray boxes contain the values between the 25th and 75th percentiles of the samples, including the median (gray line). Lines extending above and below each box symbolize data within 1.5 times the interquartile range (outliers are displayed with a +). The width of the boxes depends on the sample size. [Figure and legend from Franke et al. 2012a.]

($p < 0.05$), suggesting structural brain changes that show the pattern of accelerated aging in the pMCI and AD groups. Regarding NO and sMCI subjects, the estimated brain age at baseline did not differ significantly from the chronological age ($p = 0.61$ in both groups).

The *BrainAGE* scores remained stable for the NO and the sMCI groups across the follow-up period of up to 4 years, but increased in the pMCI and AD groups, suggesting additional acceleration in brain aging in the pMCI and AD groups. The fit of the longitudinal changes in *BrainAGE* resulted in the following changing rates (*BrainAGE* years per follow-up year): NO = 0.12, sMCI = 0.07, pMCI = 1.05, and AD = 1.51 (Figure 3.4). These rates differed among the groups ($F = 23.1$, $p < 0.001$), with post-hoc t-tests showing significant differences between NO/sMCI vs. pMCI/AD ($p < 0.05$). At the last MRI scan of each subject, the *BrainAGE* scores also differed among the groups ($F = 44.0$, $p < 0.001$), resulting in the following: NO = –0.06 years, sMCI = –0.38 years, pMCI = 8.96 years, and AD = 9.02 years (Figure 3.3B). Again,

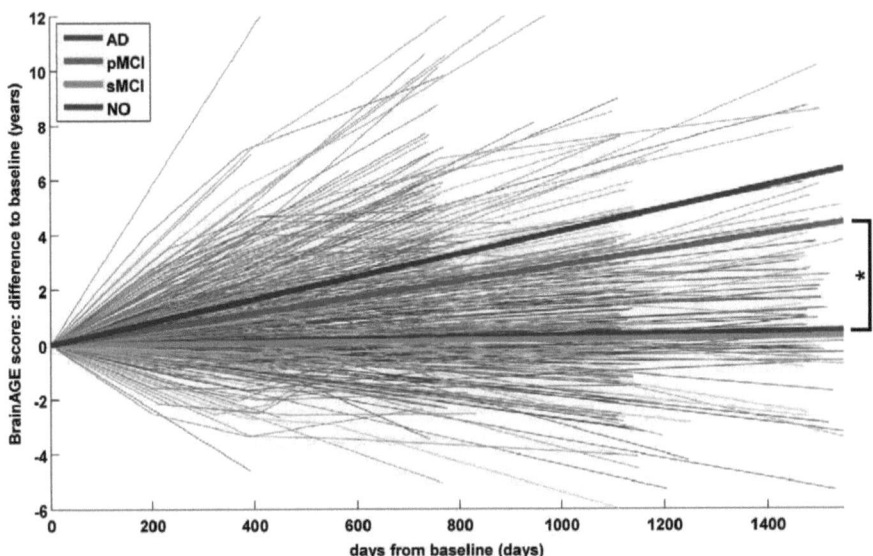

Figure 3.4: Longitudinal changes in *BrainAGE* scores for NO, sMCI, pMCI, and AD. Thin lines represent individual changes in *BrainAGE* over time; thick lines indicate estimated average changes for each group. Post-hoc t-tests showed significant differences in the longitudinal *BrainAGE* changes between NO/sMCI vs. pMCI/AD ($p < 0.05$). [Figure and legend from Franke et al. 2012a.]

post-hoc t-tests showed significant differences between NO/sMCI vs. pMCI/AD ($p < 0.05$). Regarding NO and sMCI subjects, the estimated brain age at baseline did not differ significantly from the chronological age ($p = 0.92$ and $p = 0.68$, respectively).

Taken together, these results suggest that the acceleration in brain aging in pMCI and AD found at baseline becomes even more accelerated during the next months and years. On the other hand, the results suggest that brain aging in NO and sMCI remained stable during the follow-up period of 4 years, showing only normal age-related atrophy. Across the whole sample, the *BrainAGE* scores at baseline were moderately correlated with cognitive functioning and clinical disease severity up to 4 years later (Table 3.3), with larger *BrainAGE* scores being related to worse cognitive functioning and more severe clinical symptoms ($r = 0.39 - -0.46$). The *BrainAGE* scores based on the

Table 3.3: Correlation coefficients between *BrainAGE* and cognitive functioning (ADAS scores) as well as disease severity (MMSE & CDR scores) for the whole test sample as well as for each diagnostic group separately.

	NO	sMCI	pMCI	AD	Whole sample
Correlation with *BrainAGE* score at baseline					
MMSE score at last scan	−0.14	0.09	−0.18	**−0.38*****	*−0.46****
CDR score at last scan	−0.04	0.03	0.13	**0.24****	*0.39****
ADAS score at last scan	−0.03	−0.24	**0.33*****	**0.31*****	*0.45****
Correlation with *BrainAGE* score at last scan					
MMSE score at last scan	−0.12	0.01	**−0.28****	**−0.46*****	*−0.55****
CDR score at last scan	0.01	−0-09	**0.20***	**0.30*****	*0.46****
ADAS score at last scan	−0.04	−0.10	**0.40*****	**0.37*****	*0.55****
Correlation with change in *BrainAGE* scores (baseline – last scan)					
MMSE change	0.09	−0.29	**−0.23***	**−0.23****	*−0.33****
CDR change	0.13	−0.27	**0.19***	**0.19***	*0.27****
ADAS change	−0.10	−0.04	**0.29****	**0.16***	*0.30****

[Notes: * $p < 0.05$, ** $p < 0.01$, *** $p < 0.001$. **Bold** type = significant correlations, *italic* type = whole sample.]

last MRI scan correlated even slightly stronger with cognitive scores and clinical severity of the last follow-up visit ($r = 0.46 - -0.55$). The changes in *BrainAGE* scores were also related to the individual changes in all of the three scores ($r = 0.27 - -0.33$). These results denote a close relationship between accelerated brain aging and prospective worsening of cognitive functioning within the whole sample, i.e., within the full variance of cognitive as well as *BrainAGE* scores.

Even more interesting, when analyzing each diagnostic group separately, we found these relationships between *BrainAGE* and cognitive as well as severity scores were only in the pMCI and AD groups, but not in sMCI and NO groups (Table 3.3). In pMCI, the strongest correlation with *BrainAGE* was found in ADAS ($r = 0.40$, $p < 0.001$), which is a rather cognitive scale. In AD, the strongest correlation with *BrainAGE* was found in MMSE ($r = -0.46$, $p < 0.001$), which is commonly used to measure disease severity in AD. These results strongly support the recent result of profound accelerated brain aging being related to disease severity, most pronounced in subjects being already diagnosed with AD, and prospective worsening of cognitive functioning, most pronounced in pMCI subjects.

3.5 Discussion

This study described and implemented a novel MRI-based biomarker, aggregating the complex, multidimensional aging pattern across the whole brain into one single value, i.e., the *BrainAGE* score that directly quantifies acceleration or deceleration in individual brain aging. The *BrainAGE* framework comprises well-established and fully automated processing of the T1-weighted MR images and allows one to combine data from different MRI scanners. With correlations between chronological age and estimated brain age of $r = 0.92$ in healthy adults, aged 20 – 86 years (Franke et al., 2010), and $r = 0.93$ in healthy children and adolescents, aged 5 – 18 years (Franke et al., 2012b), the *BrainAGE* framework has proved to be a straightforward method of accurately and reliably estimating brain age with minimal preprocessing and parameter optimization.

Most remarkably, although brain maturation in childhood as well as brain aging in late life comprise very complex, multidimensional, and highly variable processes (Good et al., 2001; Lebel and Beaulieu, 2011; Lenroot and Giedd, 2006; Wilke and Holland, 2003), the confidence intervals of estimated brain age did not change as a function of age (Franke et al., 2010, 2012b). This underlines the great potential of the approach to correctly capture the multi-dimensional characteristics of the different maturational and aging processes occurring in childhood and old age, respectively.

Here, the *BrainAGE* framework was trained with whole-brain structural MRI data of about 560 healthy subjects, aged 20 – 86 years. The model of healthy brain aging was then applied to new data samples. First, the stability of individual *BrainAGE* scores was examined. With ICCs 0.93 and 0.90 between the *BrainAGE* scores calculated from two shortly delayed scans on the same MRI scanner and on different 1.5T and 3.0T scanners, respectively, the *BrainAGE* framework proved its ability to provide reliable estimates.

The sample-specific offsets that emerged in the estimation of *BrainAGE* scores seem to depend on the kind of MRI scanner used, its field-strength, the scanning sequences, and other sample-specific parameters. Therefore, the influences of varying image quality and segmentation quality in training and test data on brain age estimation quality limit the reliability of the proposed method and should thus be carefully controlled in future studies as well as analyzed further within even larger samples. But since these offsets proved to be systematic in all subjects within the same sample, it can be easily controlled for by a linear shift. When quantifying brain aging and comparing *BrainAGE* in different clinical samples, one should include samples of healthy subjects in order to control for potential sample-specific and / or MRI-scanner-specific offsets in the estimated scores. There is no need to include control subjects to correct for potential offsets when examining only the relation between *BrainAGE* and other measures or the difference between brain aging in two subsamples of the same sample. Here, the *BrainAGE* framework is robust and can furthermore be applied to and generalized across different scanners. These results are in line with Klöppel et al. (2008b), indicating that the effect of the scanner is suffciently different from that of aging processes.

Regarding the relevance within the clinical context, the *BrainAGE* approach again proved its potential to indicate accelerated brain aging based on structural MRI data. Subjects with AD and subjects with MCI who converted to AD and cognitively declined within 3 years of follow-up (pMCI) exhibited significantly larger baseline *BrainAGE* scores compared to control subjects and those with MCI who remained cognitively stable (sMCI). Further, the *BrainAGE* framework even proved its capability of recognizing accelerated brain atrophy in a longitudinal design. Already starting with a higher baseline

BrainAGE score of about 6 to 7 years in pMCI and AD, brain aging accelerates even more during follow-up, at the speed of 1 additional year in brain atrophy per follow-up year in pMCI subjects and 1.5 additional years in brain atrophy per follow-up year in AD patients. This accumulated to a mean *BrainAGE* score of about 9 years at the last scan in both groups, with mean follow-up durations of 2.6 years for pMCI and 1.7 years for AD. Compared to that, sMCI and healthy control subjects did not show any deviations from healthy brain aging at baseline or at follow-up. These results are in line with recent studies that showed increased GM atrophy of approximately 2% per year in AD (Anderson et al., 2012), accelerated changes in whole brain volume in MCI (Driscoll et al., 2009), acceleration in atrophy rates as subjects progress from MCI to AD (Jack et al., 2008), and greater GM loss in certain regions in pMCI subjects (Chételat et al., 2005; Desikan et al., 2008; Leow et al., 2009; McDonald et al., 2012; Sluimer et al., 2009). Furthermore, our results also support the assumption of AD being a form of or at least being associated with accelerated aging (Cao et al., 2010; Driscoll et al., 2009; Dukart et al., 2011; Jones et al., 2011; Saetre et al., 2011; Spulber et al., 2010).

Additionally, the individual *BrainAGE* scores were clearly related to measures of severity of clinical disease, most pronounced in subjects already diagnosed as AD, as well as cognitive functioning, most pronounced in MCI subjects converting to AD within the next 3 years. Even more interestingly and clinically valuable, the *BrainAGE* scores estimated at baseline were already moderately correlated to the prospective worsening of cognitive functioning within the next 3 years. Cognitive decline was recently found to progressively accelerate years before being diagnosed as AD (Wilson et al., 2011), and be correlated with the atrophy rates in specified brain regions (Desikan et al., 2008). Our results support the suggested relationship between progressive acceleration in brain aging and rate of change in cognitive functioning as well as clinical severity in pMCI and AD during follow-up.

Furthermore, we could even show a distinct pattern of accelerated brain aging in pMCI subjects being more closely related to the worsening of higher cognitive functions, but slightly less with disease severity, whereas in AD patients accelerated brain aging was more closely related to disease severity and slightly less with the worsening of higher cognitive functions. Regarding NO and sMCI subjects, a ceiling effect was observed as well as a slightly lower variance within the cognitive scores. This may be mainly due to the fact that the scales analyzed in this study were used specifically to identify clinical disease severity as well as deterioration in cognitive functioning in the ADNI sample. Future work should further explore the relationship between *BrainAGE* and cognitive functioning with cognitive scales that are more appropriate to capture healthy cognitive aging.

In conclusion, the *BrainAGE* framework demonstrated its potential to reliably indicate accelerated brain aging. Since an additional increase in *BrainAGE* scores as well as profound relationships to disease severity and prospective worsening of cognitive functions were found in pMCI and AD during follow-up, the validity of individual *BrainAGE* scores indicating accelerated brain aging is further strengthened. Future work should demonstrate the applicability of the *BrainAGE* method on a single subject level in order to indicate early on those people at risk for converting to AD. Recently, we already demonstrated the capability of the *BrainAGE* approach to work on a single subject level by classifying subjects as either children (age range 5 – 10 years) or adolescents (age range 13 – 18 years), based on their estimated brain age, with 97% accuracy (sensitivity = 98%, specificity = 96%; Franke et al., 2012b).

The implication of these results is that this approach could potentially lead to improved identification of people at risk of faster degradation of brain structure and function and potential risk for AD, thus contributing to an early diagnosis of neurodegenerative diseases, and facilitate early treatment or a preventative intervention. Depending on the availability of subject data, future explorations could include applying this approach to several risk factors for accelerated brain aging and dementia, like diabetes (de Bresser et al., 2010; van Elderen et al., 2010), the metabolic syndrome (Solfrizzi et al., 2011), or other lifestyle factors (Chen et al., 2009; Clarke, 2006; Scarmeas et al., 2009; Solfrizzi et al., 2008), to predict the severity of clinical symptoms or the rate of cognitive decline, to differentiate between different kinds of dementia (e.g., fronto-temporal dementia), and to evaluate the therapeutic effect of drugs or other treatment modalities. Additionally, since individual quality of life is increasingly being suggested as a crucial outcome variable for health-improving and preventive interventions in old age (Garratt et al., 2002; Martin et al., 2012), it may be enlightening to integrate the *BrainAGE* approach into the recently presented "functional quality of life" (*f*QOL) model (Martin et al., 2012). This model determines the quality of life with a dynamic approach, allowing the testing of the complex relations between individual functionality judgments (e.g., individual resources, activities, central life domains) and how these relations can be adapted to stabilize or increase individual *f*QOL. Moreover, the *f*QOL can be applied to compare between and within subjects across the lifespan. Hence, future work may examine the functional value of individual *BrainAGE* scores and its complex interactions with *f*QOL-determining variables such as subjective representations as well as evaluations of cognitive performance (e.g., memory) in order to finally determine individuals' overall quality of life.

Consequently, in the future this novel *BrainAGE* approach may prove clinically valuable in detecting both normal and abnormal brain aging, providing important prognostic information.[15]

---

[15] **Acknowledgments:** Data collection and sharing for this project was funded by the Alzheimer's Disease Neuroimaging Initiative (ADNI, National Institutes of Health Grant U01 AG024904; http://adni.loni.ucla.edu). ADNI is funded by the National Institute on Aging, the National Institute of Biomedical Imaging and Bioengineering, and through generous contributions from the following organizations: Abbott; Alzheimer's Association; Alzheimer's Drug Discovery Foundation; Amorfix

Chapter 4.

Advanced *BrainAGE* in older adults with type 2 diabetes mellitus [16]

4.1 Abstract

Aging alters brain structure and function and diabetes mellitus (DM) may accelerate this process. This study investigated the effects of type 2 DM on individual brain aging as well as the relationships between individual brain aging, risk factors and functional measures. To differentiate a pattern of brain atrophy that deviates from normal brain aging, we used the novel *BrainAGE* approach, which determines the complex multidimensional aging pattern within the whole brain by applying established kernel regression methods to anatomical brain MRIs. The *"Brain Age Gap Estimation"* (*BrainAGE*) score was then calculated as the difference between chronological age and estimated brain age. 185 subjects (98 with type 2 DM) completed an MRI at 3.0T, laboratory and clinical assessments. Twenty-five subjects (12 with type 2 DM) also completed a follow-up visit after 3.8 ± 1.5 years.

The estimated brain age of DM subjects was 4.6 ± 7.2 years greater than their chronological age (p = 0.0001), whereas within the control group, esti-

---

Life Sciences Ltd.; AstraZeneca; Bayer HealthCare; BioClinica, Inc.; Biogen Idec Inc.; Bristol-Myers Squibb Company; Eisai Inc.; Elan Pharmaceuticals Inc.; Eli Lilly and Company; F. Hoffmann-La Roche Ltd. and its affiliated company Genentech, Inc.; GE Healthcare; Innogenetics, N. V.; IXICO Ltd.; Janssen Alzheimer Immunotherapy Research Development, LLC.; Johnson Johnson Pharmaceutical Research Development LLC.; Medpace, Inc.; Merck Co., Inc.; Meso Scale Diagnostics, LLC.; Novartis Pharmaceuticals Corporation; Pfizer Inc.; Servier; Synarc Inc.; and Takeda Pharmaceutical Company. The Canadian Institutes of Health Research provides funds to support ADNI clinical sites in Canada. Private sector contributions are facilitated by the Foundation for the National Institutes of Health (www.fnih.org). The grantee organization is the Northern California Institute for Research and Education, and the study is coordinated by the Alzheimer's Disease Cooperative Study at the University of California, San Diego. ADNI data are disseminated by the Laboratory for Neurolmaging at the University of California, Los Angeles. This research was also supported by NIH grants P30 AG010129 and K01 AG030514.

[16] Research article [published as: Franke, K., Gaser, C., Manor, B., and Novak, V. (2013). Advanced *BrainAGE* in older adults with type 2 diabetes mellitus. Frontiers in Aging Neuroscience, 5(90):doi: 10.3389/fnagi.2013.00090.]

mated brain age was similar to chronological age. As compared to baseline, the average *BrainAGE* scores of DM subjects increased by 0.2 years per follow-up year ($p = 0.034$), whereas the *BrainAGE* scores of controls did not change between baseline and follow-up. At baseline, across all subjects, higher *BrainAGE* scores were associated with greater smoking and alcohol consumption, higher tumor necrosis factor alpha (TNFα) levels, lower verbal fluency scores and more severe depression. Within the DM group, higher *BrainAGE* scores were associated with longer diabetes duration ($r = 0.31$, $p = 0.019$) and increased fasting blood glucose levels ($r = 0.34$, $p = 0.025$).

In conclusion, type 2 DM is independently associated with structural changes in the brain that reflect advanced aging. The *BrainAGE* approach may thus serve as a clinically relevant biomarker for the detection of abnormal patterns of brain aging associated with type 2 DM.

4.2 Introduction

The global prevalence of type 2 diabetes mellitus (DM) is projected to rise sharply over the coming decades. Individuals aged 65 years and older have a particularly high risk of developing diabetes complications, due to the combination of both modifiable (i.e., lifestyle) and non-modifiable risk factors (Zimmet et al., 2001). Within this population, type 2 DM has been linked to increased brain atrophy (Araki et al., 1994; de Bresser et al., 2010; Last et al., 2007; Novak et al., 2011; Schmidt et al., 2004; van Elderen et al., 2010), impaired cognitive function (Reijmer et al., 2011) and increased risk of depression (Ali et al., 2006; Anderson et al., 2001) and dementia, including both vascular dementia and Alzheimer's disease (AD; Biessels et al., 2006; Cheng et al., 2012; Janson et al., 2004; Tan et al., 2011; Velayudhan et al., 2010; Xu et al., 2004).

Chronic hyperglycemia is associated with vascular disease and neurotoxicity leading to neuronal damage (Tomlinson and Gardiner, 2008). Within the brain, hyperglycemia appears to induce structural abnormalities resembling the progressive, widespread atrophy often associated with biological aging (Biessels et al., 2006; Gispen and Biessels, 2000). Moreover, within the DM population, such generalized atrophy may be detected at an earlier age (Araki et al., 1994). Clinical manifestations of DM-related brain abnormalities include worse functional status (Biessels et al., 2006; Stewart and Liolitsa, 1999), deficits in cognition (i.e., verbal memory, mental flexibility, and processing speed; Cheng et al., 2012; Gispen and Biessels, 2000), and depression (Heuser, 2002; Katon et al., 2012; Wolkowitz et al., 2010, 2011). As such, recognition and quantification of subtle deviations from aging-related brain atrophy may afford prospective identification and subsequent treatment of patients with DM who are at risk for clinically-significant functional decline.

Based on the widespread but well-ordered brain tissue loss that occurs with healthy aging into senescence (Good et al., 2001), we previously proposed a modeling approach to identify abnormal aging-related brain atrophy that may precede the onset of clinical symptoms. We introduced a novel *BrainAGE* approach (Franke et al., 2010, 2012b) based on a database of single time-point structural magnetic resonance imaging (MRI) data that aggregates the complex, multidimensional aging patterns across the whole brain to one single value, i.e. the estimated brain age (Figure 1.4A; page 21). Consequently, subtle deviations in "normal" brain atrophy can be directly quantified in terms of years by analyzing only one standard MRI scan per subject (Figure 1.4B; page 21). Recently, we demonstrated that the *BrainAGE* approach enables the identification of advanced brain aging in subjects with mild cognitive impairment and AD, and observed profound relationships between *BrainAGE*, disease severity, prospective worsening of cognitive functions (Franke et al., 2012a), conversion to AD (Gaser et al., 2013), as well as certain health and lifestyle markers (e.g., the metabolic syndrome; Franke et al., 2013b).

In this study, we implemented the *BrainAGE* method to quantify the effects of type 2 DM on individual brain aging in non-demented older adults. We further explored the relationships between individual brain aging and clinically significant lifestyle risk factors (i.e., smoking duration, alcohol intake), clinical laboratory data (i.e., fasting blood glucose level as a potential indicator of hyperglycemia, tumor necrosis factor alpha (TNFα) as a potential indicator of persistent inflammation), and common clinical outcomes (i.e., cognition, depression). We hypothesized that type 2 DM is associated with greater *BrainAGE* scores, and that clinically significant risk factors additionally contribute to this process. We also hypothesized that those individuals with greater *BrainAGE* scores would also exhibit worse outcomes related to cognition and depression.

4.3 Research design and methods
4.3.1 Subjects

To train the age estimation framework, we used MRI data of 561 healthy subjects (250 male) from the publicly accessible IXI cohort[17] (data downloaded in September 2011) aged 20 – 86 years (mean (SD) = 48.6 (16.5) years; for more sample details see Franke et al., 2010).

The current *BrainAGE* analyses were conducted using existing records of 185 subjects (98 with diagnosed type 2 DM; Table 4.1), who previously participated in studies within the Syncope and Falls in the Elderly (SAFE) Laboratory at the Beth Israel Deaconess Medical Center (BIDMC). A subset of these subjects (n = 25, 12 with type 2 DM; Table 4.2) also completed a follow-up MR scan after an average of 3.8 years (SD = 1.5).

Participants were recruited consecutively via advertisement in the local community and provided informed consent as approved by the Institutional

---

[17] www.brain-development.org

Table 4.1: Demographic and clinical variables of the cross-sectional control and type 2 DM groups.

	Non-diabetic control group	Type 2 DM group	p
No. subjects	87	98	n.s.
Males / Females	41 / 46	53 / 45	n.s.
Age mean (years)	65.3 (8.5)	64.6 (8.1)	n.s.
Hypertension (yes / no)	22 / 65	56 / 42	*
Diabetes duration (years)	–	11.3 (9.3)	–
GM volume (ml)	528.9 (63.5)	519.0 (52.3)	n.s.
WM volume (ml)	540.2 (78.3)	536.2 (90.8)	n.s.
Total brain volume (ml)	1347.7 (147.2)	1338.1 (146.2)	n.s.
BMI (kg/m^2)	25.4 (3.7)	28.8 (4.8)	***
Smoking duration (years)	9.4 (15.1)	10.9 (14.6)	n.s.
Alcohol intake (dose / week)	2.0 (3.3)	5.1 (14.3)	n.s.
Non-fasting blood glucose (mg/dL)	82.0 (13.2)	124.0 (56.4)	***
Fasting blood glucose (Visit 2)	86.7 (13.6)	110.6 (32.4)	n.s.
TNFα (pg/mL)	1.6 (0.7)	1.6 (0.5)	n.s.
Verbal fluency (T-score)	50.0 (10.1)	39.5 (12.8)	***
Geriatric Depression Scale (total score)	3.8 (4.8)	6.4 (6.4)	n.s.

[*Notes:* Data are means ± (SD) unless otherwise indicated. p denotes between-group comparisons. * $p < 0.05$, *** $p < 0.001$.]

Review Board. Controls were required to have normal fasting glucose, but had a similar distribution of risk factors. All participants were screened with a medical history and physical and laboratory examinations. Participants with DM were treated with insulin, oral glucose-control agents (sulfonylurea, second generation agents or their combinations), or diet only. Several participants in each group were treated for hypertension and / or hypercholesterolemia. Excluded were participants with type 1 DM, a history of stroke, myocardial infarction within 6 months, and other clinically important cardiac diseases, arrhythmias, significant nephropathy, kidney or liver transplant, renal or congestive heart failure, carotid artery stenosis (over 50% by medical history and MR angiography), neurological or other systemic disorders; claustrophobia, metal implants, pacemakers, arterial stents incompatible with MRI.

Table 4.2: Demographic and clinical variables of the longitudinal subsample.

		Non-diabetic control group	Type 2 DM group	p
No. subjects		13	12	n.s.
Males / Females		5 / 8	4 / 8	n.s.
Hypertension (yes / no)		2 /11	7 / 5	n.s.
Baseline	Age mean (years)	69.9 (5.5)	63.3 (6.9)	*
	GM volume (ml)	501.6 (62.5)	439.1 (47.4)	n.s.
	WM volume (ml)	528.7 (84.1)	554.5 (76.6)	n.s.
	Total brain volume (ml)	1308.1 (143.9)	1302.0 (150.8)	n.s.
Follow-up	Age mean (years)	73.9 (5.7)	66.8 (6.7)	**
	GM volume (ml)	511.7 (63.6)	505.1 (47.7)	n.s.
	WM volume (ml)	522.9 (65.0)	533.7 (108.8)	n.s.
	Total brain volume (ml)	1306.3 (127.6)	1303.5 (161.8)	n.s.

[*Notes:* Data are means ± (SD) unless otherwise indicated. *p* denotes between-group comparisons. * *p* < 0.05, ** *p* < 0.01.]

All participants were admitted to the Clinical Research Center for an overnight stay. Laboratory chemistries were collected after overnight fasting, and MRI was done before noon. Functional clinical outcomes were acquired through a battery of neuropsychological tests, including assessments for learning and memory, depression, and physical function.

In order to quantify the relationship between *BrainAGE* scores, life-style risk factors and clinical outcomes, the following data were extracted: body mass index (BMI), smoking duration, alcohol intake, non-fasting blood glucose levels, parameters of diabetes control (duration, fasting blood glucose levels), common clinical outcomes (i.e., verbal fluency, more specifically "semantic fluency", requiring the generation of exemplars of the category "animals"; Harrison et al., 2000; Fisher et al., 2004) and depression as measured with the Geriatric Depression Scale (GDS; Yesavage, 1988), and inflammation markers (TNFα).

4.3.2 Magnetic resonance imaging (MRI)

All studies were performed within the Center for Advanced MR Imaging at the BIDMC on the same 3.0 Tesla GE HDx MRI scanner using a quadrature and phase array head coils (GE Medical Systems, Milwaukee, WI). Anatomical images were acquired using 3-D magnetization prepared rapid gradient echo (MP-RAGE) ($T_R / T_E / T_I$ = 7.8 / 3.1 / 600 ms, 3.0 mm slice thickness, 52 slices, bandwidth = 122 Hz per pixel, flip angle = 10°, 24 cm x 24 cm FOV, 256 x 192 matrix size) and fluid attenuated inversion recovery (FLAIR) ($T_R / T_E / T_I$ = 11000 / 161 / 2250 ms, 5 mm slice thickness, 30 slices, bandwidth = 122 Hz per pixel, flip angle = 90°, 24 cm x 24 cm FOV, 256 x 160 matrix size) sequences.

4.3.3 Preprocessing of MRI data and data reduction

Preprocessing of the T1-weighted images was done using the SPM8 package[18] and the VBM8 toolbox[19], running under MATLAB. All T1-weighted images were corrected for bias-field inhomogeneities, then spatially normalized and segmented into gray matter (GM), white matter (WM), and cerebrospinal fluid (CSF) within the same generative model (Ashburner and Friston, 2005). The segmentation procedure was extended by accounting for partial volume effects (Tohka et al., 2004), by applying adaptive maximum a posteriori estimations (Rajapakse et al., 1997), and by using a hidden Markov random field model (Cuadra et al., 2005; Gaser, 2009). The images were processed with affine registration and smoothed with 8 mm full-width-at-half-maximum (FWHM) smoothing kernels. Spatial resolution was set to 8 mm. For further data reduction, principal component analysis (PCA) was performed on the training sample with subsequently applying the estimated transformation pa-

---

[18] www.fil.ion.ucl.ac.uk/spm
[19] http://dbm.neuro.uni-jena.de

rameters to the test sample. PCA was done using the "MATLAB Toolbox for Dimensionality Reduction"[20], running under MATLAB.

4.3.4 Age estimation framework

The *BrainAGE* framework utilizes a machine-learning pattern recognition method, namely relevance vector regression (RVR; Tipping, 2001). It was recently developed to estimate individual brain ages based on T1-weighted images (Franke et al., 2010). In general, the model is trained with preprocessed whole brain structural MRI data of the training sample (here: the IXI sample). Subsequently, the brain age of each test subject can be estimated using the individual tissue-classified MRI data, aggregating the complex, multidimensional aging pattern across the whole brain into one single value (Figure 1.4A; page 21). The difference between estimated and true chronological age will reveal the individual *"Brain Age Gap Estimation"* (*BrainAGE*) score. Consequently, the *BrainAGE* score directly quantifies the amount of acceleration or deceleration of brain aging. For example, if a 70 years old individual has a *BrainAGE* score of +5 years, this means that this individual shows the typical atrophy pattern of a 75 year old individual (Figure 1.4B; page 21). Recent work has demonstrated that this method provides reliable and stable estimates (Franke et al., 2012a). Specifically, the *BrainAGE* scores calculated from two shortly delayed scans on the same MRI scanner, as well as on separate 1.5T and 3.0T scanners, produced intraclass correlation coefficients (ICC) of 0.93 and 0.90, respectively.

Within this study, the *BrainAGE* framework was applied using the linear combination of preprocessed (as described in the section 4.3.3) GM and WM images. For training the model as well as for predicting individual brain ages, we used "The Spider"[21], a freely available toolbox running under MATLAB. For

---
[20] http://ict.ewi.tudelft.nl/~lvandermaaten/Home.html
[21] www.kyb.mpg.de/bs/people/spider/main.html

an illustration of the most important features (i.e., the importance of voxel locations for regression with age) that were used by the RVR to model normal brain aging and more detailed information please refer to Figure 2.5 (page 41).

4.3.5 Statistical analysis

Descriptive statistics were used to summarize all variables. Demographic and laboratory data were compared between the control and the DM groups using analysis of variance (ANOVA) for continuous variables or Kruskal-Wallis tests for categorical variables and variables that were not normally distributed. Normality was tested using Shapiro-Wilk tests. Cross-sectionally, within-group differences between estimated brain age and biological age were tested using Student's t-test.

The effect of DM on *BrainAGE* was determined with ANOVA. The dependent variable was the *BrainAGE* score. Model effects included group (i.e., DM & non-DM controls), hypertension (i.e., with / without hypertension) and gender.

Relationships between *BrainAGE* and clinical parameters were then analyzed in the whole sample (i.e., DM and non-DM subjects together), controlling for age, gender, and diabetes duration (with diabetes duration = 0 years for non-DM controls). As not all subjects had values for all clinical variables, univariate correlation analyses were used (instead of multivariate models) to assess the relationship between *BrainAGE* and distinguished lifestyle measures (i.e. BMI, smoking duration, alcohol intake), clinical laboratory data (i.e., fasting blood glucose level, TNFα), and functional measures (i.e., T-score for verbal fluency, total GDS score for depression). In order to control for covariates, Pearson's pairwise correlation were used for normally distributed variables, and Spearman's correlations were used for variables that are not normally distributed, with adjustment for age, gender and diabetes duration (right-tailed for verbal fluency, left-tailed for all others). To control for multiple comparisons, Bonferoni-Holm correction (Holm, 1979) was applied, adjusting the p-value for the number of variables analyzed (i.e., 7).

The effect of diabetes-status within the relationships between *BrainAGE* and lifestyle parameters, clinical laboratory data and outcome measures were investigated by performing analysis of covariance (ANCOVA). Each specific ANCOVA included all those subjects who were measured in each specific clinical variable, sub-grouped by DM. Since fasting blood glucose levels were provided for only three non-DM control subjects, this variable was excluded from this analysis. For all other variables, the model fitted separate lines for both groups, thus allowing the intercept as well as the slopes to vary between both groups.

To further explore the relationship between *BrainAGE* and clinical parameters, the whole sample was divided into quartiles for each of the significantly related lifestyle measures (i.e., smoking duration, alcohol intake), clinical laboratory data (i.e., fasting blood glucose level, TNFα), and outcome measures (i.e., verbal fluency, depression). To illustrate the relationships between individual brain aging and extreme levels in each of these variables, the *BrainAGE* scores in the 1st quartile (lowest 25% of values) of each lifestyle and functionality measure were tested against the *BrainAGE* scores in 4th quartile (highest 25% of values) of each lifestyle and functionality measure, using one-tailed t-tests (right-tailed for verbal fluency, left-tailed for all others). Similar, Bonferroni-Holm-adjusted p-values were used to determine significance. Within the subsample that completed two MRI scans, the longitudinal changes in individual *BrainAGE* scores were fitted against time between both scans with a multivariate linear regression model. *BrainAGE* scores at baseline and follow-up visit, as well as longitudinal changes in *BrainAGE* were compared between both groups using ANOVA.

The Shapiro-Wilk test was performed using JMP 9.0.[22] All other testing was performed using MATLAB 7.11.[23]

4.4 Results
4.4.1 Group characteristics

All variables except diabetes duration, BMI, alcohol intake and GDS scores were normally distributed. Age, gender, GM, WM and total brain volumes did not differ between groups (Table 4.1). The DM group had higher BMI ($p < 0.0001$), higher non-fasting blood glucose levels ($p < 0.0001$), greater prevalence of hypertension ($p < 0.05$), and worse performance in verbal fluency ($p < 0.0001$) than controls (Table 4.1).

4.4.2 Cross-sectional *BrainAGE* analyses

Although brain volumes did not differ between the groups, the DM subjects had significantly higher *BrainAGE* scores than controls ($F = 17.2$, $p = 0.0001$; Figure 4.1). Additionally, *BrainAGE* scores did not correlate to brain volumes (Figure 4.2). Within the control group, estimated brain age was similar to chronological age ($t_{(0.975,86)} = 0.0$, $p = 1.0$). In DM subjects, however, the average *BrainAGE* score was 4.6 years (SD = 7.2 years); i.e., their estimated brain age was 4.6 years greater than their chronological age ($t_{(0.975,97)} = 6.4$, $p = 0.0001$). Additionally, within the DM group, those with longer diabetes duration had higher *BrainAGE* scores ($r = 0.31$, $p = 0.019$). This relationship was independent of age, gender, and duration of hypertension history.

Across all subjects, *BrainAGE* scores were higher in males as compared to females ($F = 7.7$, $p = 0.006$). There were no effects for hypertension ($F = 0.0$, $p = 0.9$), or any interaction (group * hypertension: $F = 0.6$, $p = 0.46$; group * gender: $F = 0.7$, $p = 0.41$; hypertension * gender: $F = 0.1$, $p = 0.79$).

---
[22] www.jmp.com
[23] www.mathworks.com

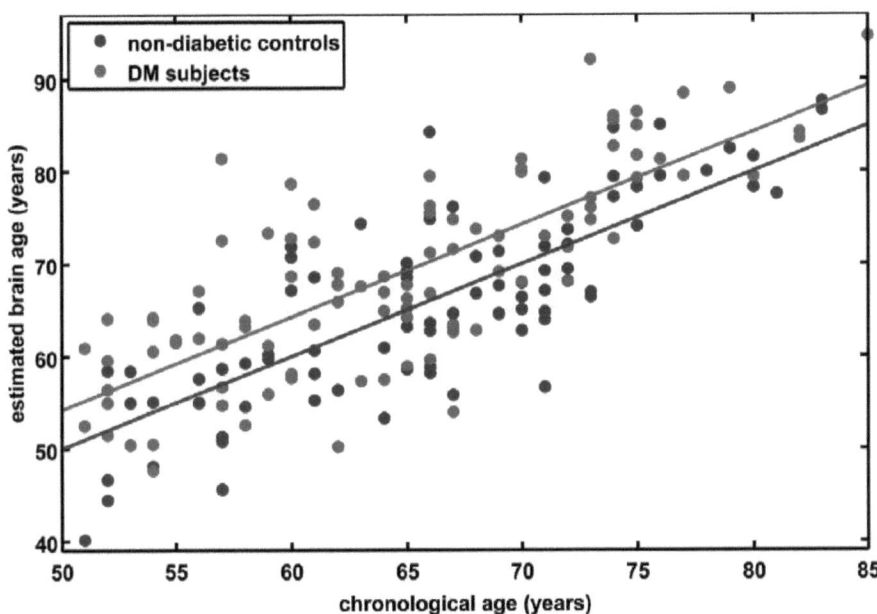

Figure 4.1: **Estimated brain age vs. chronological age for controls and subjects with type 2 DM.** The *BrainAGE* scores (i.e., the difference between the estimated and the chronological age) differed between groups, with mean (± SD) *BrainAGE* scores of 0.0 ± 6.7 years in healthy controls (blue) and 4.6 ± 7.2 years in type 2 DM subjects (red; $p < 0.0001$). [Figure and legend from Franke et al. 2013a.]

Across all subjects, higher *BrainAGE* scores were significantly correlated with lifestyle factors, i.e. increased duration of smoking ($r = 0.20$, $p = 0.007$) and greater alcohol consumption ($r = 0.24$, $p = 0.001$), as well as clinical laboratory data, i.e. higher fasting blood glucose ($r = 0.34$, $p = 0.025$) and TNFα ($r = 0.29$, $p = 0.01$) levels. Higher *BrainAGE* scores were also correlated with lower verbal fluency ($r = -0.25$, $p = 0.006$) and higher depression scores ($r = 0.23$, $p = 0.012$). All correlations were independent of age, gender, and diabetes duration.

Additionally, ANCOVAs were performed to investigate the effects of DM status on the relationships between *BrainAGE* scores and distinguished lifestyle factors, clinical variables, and outcome measures. Although *BrainAGE*

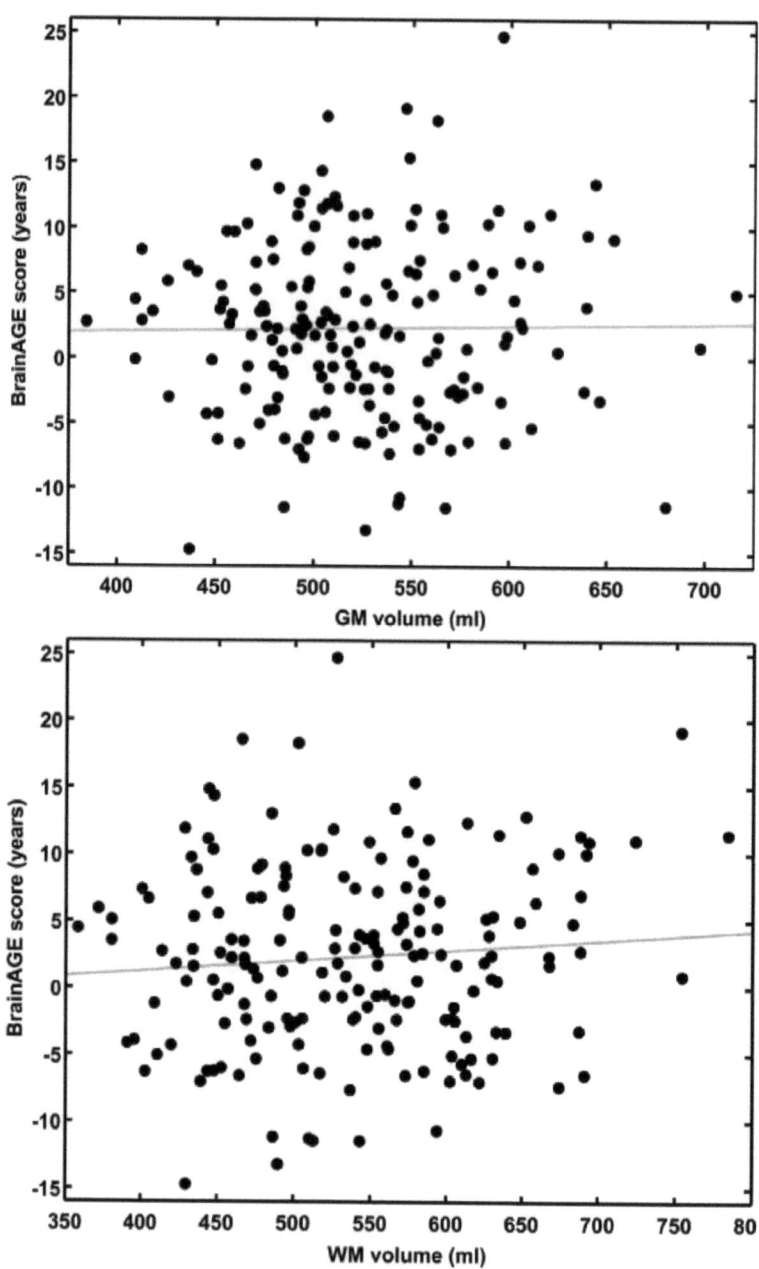

Figure 4.2: *BrainAGE* scores plotted against GM and WM volumes for all subjects. *BrainAGE* scores did not correlate to either GM (*top*; $r = 0.02$, $p = 0.81$) or WM volumes (*bottom*; $r = 0.09$, $p = 0.20$). [Figure and legend from Franke et al. 2013a.]

scores were generally higher in DM subjects, higher *BrainAGE* scores were also related to increased smoking duration ($F = 5.13$, $p < 0.05$), increased alcohol intake ($F = 7.63$, $p < 0.01$), increased TNFα ($F = 6.24$, $p < 0.05$), decreased verbal fluency ($F = 4.07$, $p < 0.05$), and increased GDS scores ($F = 7.17$, $p < 0.01$) in DM subjects as well as in non-DM controls (Table 4.3, Figure 4.3).

To exemplarily quantify the relationship between brain atrophy and lifestyle factors, clinical laboratory data and functionality, the *BrainAGE* scores of subjects with the lowest values in those measures (i.e., 1st quartile) versus subjects with the highest values in those measures (i.e., 4th quartile) were contrasted (Table 4.4, Figure 4.4). These analyses resulted in significant differences in *BrainAGE* of 3.4 years for smoking duration ($p = 0.004$), 4.1 years for alcohol intake ($p = 0.003$), 5.5 years for fasting blood glucose ($p = 0.02$), 5.4 years for TNFα ($p = 0.006$), 5.6 years for verbal fluency ($p = 0.001$), and 5.4 years for depression scores ($p = 0.002$).

4.4.3 Longitudinal *BrainAGE* analyses

A subsample of 25 subjects (12 DM subjects and 13 controls) completed a

Table 4.3: ANCOVA results for *BrainAGE* scores and distinguished variables.

	Model						Coefficient estimates			
	Group		Variable value		Group x Value		Intercept		Slope	
	F	p	F	p	F	p	t	p	t	p
BMI	17.4	**0.0001**	0.02	0.89	2.4	0.12	0.94	0.35	0.36	0.39
Smoking duration	21.4	**0.0001**	5.13	**0.02**	0.0	0.97	2.60	**0.01**	2.26	**0.02**
Alcohol intake	11.8	**0.0007**	7.63	**0.006**	6.82	**0.009**	2.13	**0.03**	3.54	**0.0005**
TNFα	11.2	**0.001**	6.24	**0.01**	0.16	0.69	1.61	0.11	2.18	**0.03**
Verbal fluency	6.28	**0.01**	4.07	**0.04**	0.06	0.80	2.79	**0.006**	1.96	*0.05*
GDS	7.12	**0.009**	7.17	**0.008**	1.46	0.23	1.47	0.14	2.94	**0.004**

[Notes: **Bold** type = significant test results.]

second MRI scan 3.8 ± 1.5 years after their baseline assessment. In this subsample, GM, WM as well as total brain volumes did not differ between groups (Table 4.2), or across time points (GM volume: $p = 0.48$; WM volume: $p = 0.58$; total brain volume: $p = 0.99$). Interestingly, however, we observed a change in *BrainAGE* over time that was dependent upon group ($F = 6.9$, $p = 0.015$; Figure 4.5). Specifically, as compared to baseline, average *BrainAGE* scores increased in DM subjects by 0.2 years per follow-up year. Within the control group, as expected, *BrainAGE* scores were similar to chronological age at baseline and follow-up and therefore did not change over time. In other words, whereas the *BrainAGE* scores of patients with DM were on average 5.1 years higher than controls at baseline ($F = 6.2$, $p = 0.020$), they were on average 5.9 years higher than controls at follow-up ($F = 5.0$, $p = 0.034$).

4.5 Discussion

This study implemented a novel MRI-based biomarker that comprises well-established and fully automated steps for processing standard T1-weighted MR images, aggregating the complex, multidimensional aging pattern across the whole brain into one single value; i.e. the *BrainAGE* score. This method has the advantage of accurately and reliably estimating brain age with minimal preprocessing and parameter optimization (Franke et al., 2010, 2012b), using a single anatomical scan. The *BrainAGE* score directly quantifies subtle deviations from the normal brain-aging pattern and may therefore provide clinically important prognostic information.

In this study, the *BrainAGE* approach was used to determine the effects of type 2 DM on brain aging. Although GM, WM and total brain volumes did not differ between groups, *BrainAGE* scores were on average 4.6 years greater in DM subjects as compared to non-DM controls. Moreover, *BrainAGE* scores

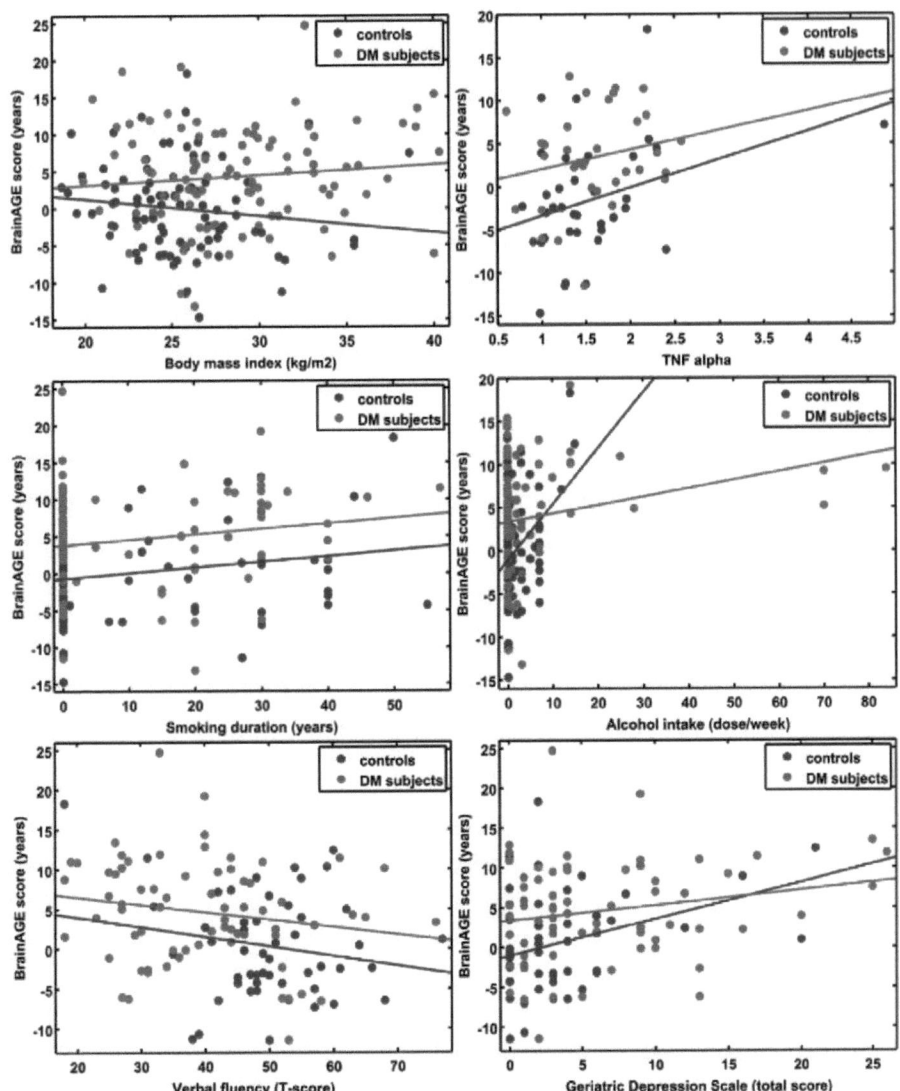

Figure 4.3: ANCOVA plots for *BrainAGE* scores and distinguished variables. *BrainAGE* scores are plotted against BMI, smoking duration, alcohol intake, TNFα, verbal fluency, and GDS scores for non-DM controls (blue) and subjects with type 2 DM (red). In both groups, higher *BrainAGE* scores were significantly related to increased smoking duration ($p < 0.05$), increased alcohol intake ($p < 0.01$), increased TNFα ($p < 0.05$), decreased verbal fluency ($p < 0.05$), and increased GDS scores ($p < 0.01$). [Figure and legend from Franke et al. 2013a.]

Table 4.4: Comparison of *BrainAGE* scores between the quartile groups in the whole sample.

	Mean (SD) *BrainAGE* score (years)				p for trend
	1st quartile	2nd quartile	3rd quartile	4th quartile	
BMI	3.04 (6.06)	0.59 (7.54)	1.68 (5.75)	3.90 (7.37)	0.29
Smoking duration	1.67 (6.43)	–	0.87 (6.51)	5.07 (7.25)	**0.012**
Alcohol intake	1.30 (6.57)	–	0.82 (5.97)	5.42 (6.07)	**0.002**
Fasting blood glucose	2.38 (7.34)	0.13 (7.67)	5.21 (4.22)	7.85 (3.02)	**0.036**
TNFα	−1.30 (6.31)	0.20 (6.64)	0.51 (7.16)	4.11 (5.75)	0.10
Verbal fluency	6.47 (6.98)	3.14 (6.92)	0.72 (5.38)	0.86 (6.63)	**0.002**
GDS	0.62 (6.56)	2.78 (7.65)	2.72 (5.37)	6.01 (5.73)	**0.015**

[Notes: **Bold** type = significant test results.]

tended to be higher in those with longer diabetes duration and higher fasting blood glucose levels, suggesting a potential link between worse glycemic control and pathologic brain atrophy. Longitudinal analyses further indicated that DM might result in greater increases in *BrainAGE* scores over time (despite no detectable change in global brain tissue volumetrics). Together, these results suggest that the *BrainAGE* score may be sensitive to subtle, glucose-mediated structural brain changes that reflect a pattern of premature brain aging (Araki et al., 1994; Biessels et al., 2006; Gispen and Biessels, 2000; van Elderen et al., 2010; Velayudhan et al., 2010; Tan et al., 2011).

This study also revealed that individual brain aging was correlated with numerous clinical outcomes. Across all subjects, and independently of diabetes duration, age and gender, those with higher *BrainAGE* scores consumed more alcohol. This observation is supported by recent studies suggesting a U-shaped relationship between alcohol consumption and cognitive impairment (Anttila et al., 2004; Solfrizzi et al., 2008). Higher *BrainAGE* scores were also linked to increased TNFα levels, which are now believed to play a central role in the pathogenesis of AD (Tobinick and Gross, 2008). To this end, those with higher *BrainAGE* scores also tended to have worse verbal fluency. Finally, those subjects with higher *BrainAGE* scores were more likely to have

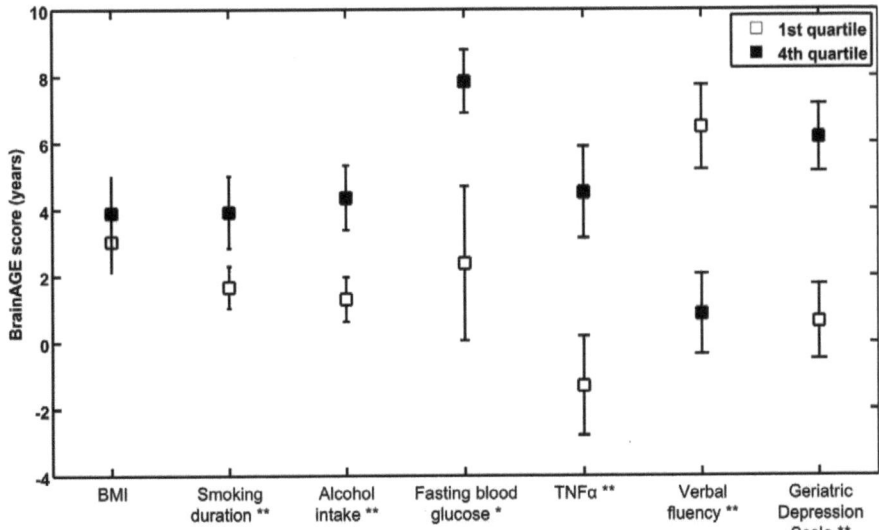

Figure 4.4: **Exemplary quartile analyses.** Mean *BrainAGE* scores in subjects with values in the 1st and 4th quartiles of distinguished variables. Error bars depict the standard error of the mean (SEM). [Figure and legend from Franke et al. 2013a.]

more severe depressive symptoms, which is in line with recent studies linking depression to both advanced brain aging (Heuser, 2002; Wolkowitz et al., 2010, 2011) as increased risk of dementia (Katon et al., 2012).

The *BrainAGE* approach was designed to recognize and indicate deviations in age-related spatiotemporal brain changes. Subjects with a high *BrainAGE* score may thus be at risk for several neurodegenerative diseases and related functional declines. Higher *BrainAGE* scores as well as profound correlations to disease severity and prospective worsening of cognitive functions have already been observed in subjects with mild cognitive impairment and AD (Franke et al., 2012a). The *BrainAGE* approach was even capable of identifying subjects who will be diagnosed with AD up to three years in advance, with each additional year in the *BrainAGE* score being associated with a 10% greater risk of developing AD (Gaser et al., 2013). As such, larger prospective trials are warranted to confirm our initial observation that type 2 DM

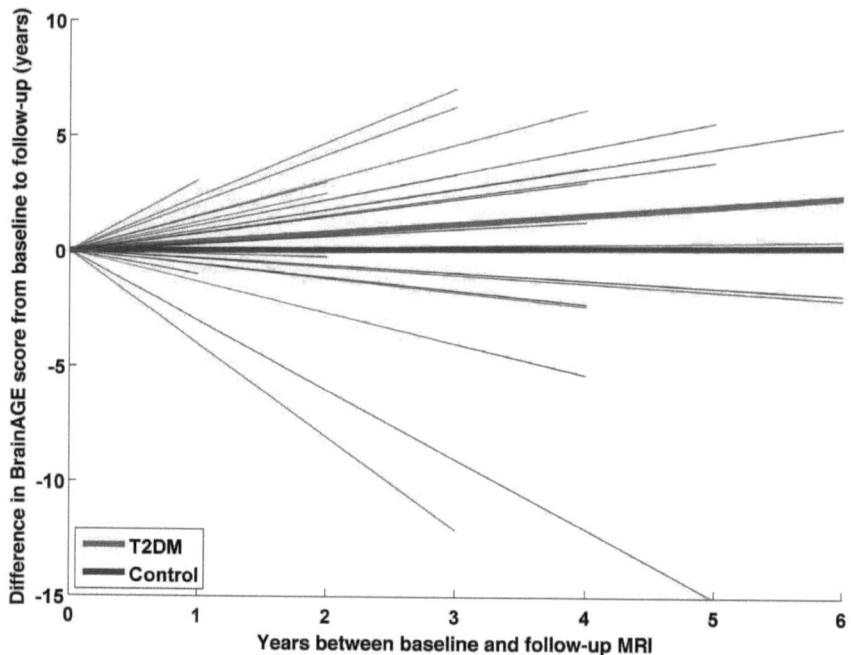

Figure 4.5: Longitudinal *BrainAGE* changes in controls and type 2 DM subjects. Longitudinal changes in *BrainAGE* scores for non-DM control subjects (blue) and type 2 DM subjects (red). Thin lines represent individual changes in *BrainAGE* over time; thick lines indicate estimated average changes for each group. The change in *BrainAGE* over time was dependent upon group ($p = 0.01$), providing preliminary longitudinal evidence that type 2 DM accelerates brain aging. [Figure and legend from Franke et al. 2013a.]

leads to premature brain aging, and to determine whether this pattern is similar to those of other neurodegenerative diseases. In future research, we aim to further explore and disentangle age- and unrelated disease-based processes of brain atrophy in neurodegenerative diseases (e.g. vascular dementia, AD) as well as its effects on *BrainAGE* estimations.

In the present study, there was considerable variance associated with individual *BrainAGE* scores, as well as intra-individual changes in *BrainAGE* scores over time. As we have previously reported (Franke et al., 2013b), and confirmed in this study, a number of nutrition, lifestyle, and health parameters likely contribute to this variance. For example, in older male adults without major disease, 39% of the inter-subject variance in *BrainAGE* was explained by the set of clinical markers under consideration, with markers of the metabolic syndrome mainly contributing to this variance (Franke et al., 2013b). As individual changes in lifestyle (e.g., smoking cessation, physical activity, intake of unsaturated fatty acids, moderate alcohol intake) were shown to lower the risk of cognitive decline and dementia (Erickson et al., 2010; Frisardi et al., 2010; Nepal et al., 2010), such lifestyle changes may be also related to a decrease in individual *BrainAGE*. Future research is therefore warranted to determine the effects of individual health and lifestyle modification, as well as improved DM control (e.g., a lowering of blood glucose levels), on longitudinal changes in individual *BrainAGE* scores.

It is of note that white matter lesions, which occur primarily due to cerebro-vascular diseases (Hadjidemetriou et al., 2008; Zhan et al., 2009), are not detected in the segmentation approach used within the *BrainAGE* analysis. Such lesions segmented as GM may therefore influence the relevance vector regression. However, as the prevalence of white matter lesions was minimal in the current cohort, it is unlikely that this limitation influenced the training of "normal brain aging". Thus, even though the current *BrainAGE* method has high test-retest reliability (Franke et al., 2012a), it may benefit from the development and implementation of segmentation methods that enable automated detection of white matter lesions even without any additional FLAIR sequence (Klöppel et al., 2011).

As not all subjects had values for all clinical variables, we were unable to utilize multivariate models to examine the relationship between *BrainAGE* and health-related outcomes, as this approach would have resulted in an extreme reduction in sample size ($n = 17$). Future studies with larger samples are therefore needed to enable multivariate analyses designed to identify the complex interactions between brain aging, lifestyle factors and clinical outcomes. Moreover, as our prospective cohort was rather small, it still remains unclear whether the presence of type 2 DM and / or lifestyle risk factors represents the cause or consequence of observed associations. Further research is therefore needed to extend our results on the longitudinal relationships between individual brain aging and miscellaneous risk factors (e.g., diabetes, lifestyle, depression) in a larger population-based sample. Furthermore, the relationship between the duration of exposure to risk factors and accelerated brain aging, and whether reversal of modifiable factors might decelerate the progression of brain aging, should be explored.

As *BrainAGE* scores are calculated from a single T1-weighted MRI per subject, using processing techniques that can be fully automated with multi-centre data, this approach may be easily implemented into clinical practice in order to encourage the identification of subtle, yet clinically-significant, changes in brain structure. With regards to type 2 DM, the implications of this study may lead to a clinical tool that identifies people at risk of faster degradation of brain structure and function and potential risk for dementias, thus contributing to an early diagnosis of neurodegenerative diseases and facilitating early treatment or preventative interventions.

Chapter 5.

BrainAGE in mild cognitive impaired patients: Predicting the conversion to Alzheimer's disease [24]

5.1 Abstract

Alzheimer's disease (AD), the most common form of dementia, shares many aspects of abnormal brain aging. We present a novel magnetic resonance imaging (MRI)-based biomarker that predicts the individual progression of mild cognitive impairment (MCI) to AD on the basis of pathological brain aging patterns. By employing kernel regression methods, the expression of normal brain-aging patterns forms the basis to estimate the brain age of a given new subject. If the estimated age is higher than the chronological age, a positive *"Brain Age Gap Estimation"* (*BrainAGE*) score indicates accelerated atrophy and is considered a risk factor for conversion to AD.

Here, the *BrainAGE* framework was applied to predict the individual brain ages of 195 subjects with MCI at baseline, of which a total of 133 developed AD during 36 months of follow-up (corresponding to a pre-test probability of 68%). The ability of the *BrainAGE* framework to correctly identify MCI-converters was compared with the performance of commonly used cognitive scales, hippocampus volume, and state-of-the-art biomarkers derived from cerebrospinal fluid (CSF). With accuracy rates of up to 81%, *BrainAGE* outperformed all cognitive scales and CSF biomarkers in predicting conversion of MCI to AD within 3 years of follow-up. Each additional year in the *BrainAGE* score was associated with a 10% greater risk of developing AD (hazard rate: 1.10 [CI: 1.07 − 1.13]). Furthermore, the post-test probability was in-

---

[24] Research article [published as: Gaser, C., Franke, K., Klöppel, S., Koutsouleris, N., Sauer, H., and Alzheimer's Disease Neuroimaging Initiative (2013). *BrainAGE* in mild cognitive impaired patients: Predicting the conversion to Alzheimer's disease. *PLoS One*, 8(6):e67346.]

creased to 90% when using baseline *BrainAGE* scores to predict conversion to AD.

The presented framework allows an accurate prediction even with multi-center data. Its fast and fully automated nature facilitates the integration into the clinical workflow. It can be exploited as a tool for screening as well as for monitoring treatment options.

5.2 Background

The global prevalence of dementia is projected to rise sharply over the coming decades. By 2050, 1 in 85 persons worldwide will be affected by Alzheimer's disease (AD), the most common form of dementia (Brookmeyer et al., 2007). Manifold pathological changes begin to develop years or decades before the onset of cognitive decline (Jack et al., 2010), including premature changes in gene expression (Cao et al., 2010; Saetre et al., 2011), accelerated age-associated changes of the default mode network (Jones et al., 2011), and most obviously, abnormal changes in brain structures already at the mild cognitive impairment (MCI) stage (Driscoll et al., 2009; Spulber et al., 2010). Additionally, atrophic regions detected in AD patients were recently found to largely overlap with those regions showing a normal age-related decline in healthy control subjects (Dukart et al., 2011).

Early detection and quantification of abnormal brain changes is important for the prospective identification and subsequent treatment of individuals at risk for cognitive decline and dementia. The best validated biomarkers for an early detection include markers of brain β-amyloid-plaque (Aβ) deposition, i.e. decreased cerebrospinal fluid (CSF) Aβ_{42} and positive Pittsburgh compound B (PiB) amyloid imaging, as well as markers of neurodegeneration, i.e. increased CSF tau, decreased fluorodeoxyglucose uptake on PET (FDG-PET), and structural magnetic resonance imaging (MRI) measures of cerebral atrophy (Jack et al., 2010). More specifically, low concentrations of CSF Aβ_{42}, associated with the formation of Aβ plaques in the brain, were found to correlate with the clinical diagnosis of AD (Clark et al., 2003; Strozyk et al., 2003), but not with rates of brain atrophy (Josephs et al., 2008). The process of Aβ-plaque accumulation begins at least 5 – 10 years (Buchhave et al., 2012) or even up to two decades before probable manifestation of clinical symptoms and conversion to AD (Jack et al., 2009), but on its own is not sufficient to cause dementia (Aizenstein et al., 2008; Jack et al., 2010; Peskind et al., 2006; Price and Morris, 1999; Price et al., 2009; Savva et al., 2009). At some point in the AD disease course accelerated neurodegeneration takes place, preceding accelerated cognitive decline (Jack et al., 2010). Although CSF tau was found to positively correlate with severity of cognitive impairment (Buchhave et al., 2012; Shaw et al., 2009), increased CSF tau is not specific for AD but seems to indicate neuronal injury and neurodegeneration in general (Hesse et al., 2001; Jack et al., 2010; Schoonenboom et al., 2012). Although brain atrophy in general is not specific for AD, MRI-detected atrophy was found to retain the closest relationship with cognitive decline (Jack et al., 2010; Vemuri et al., 2009a,b) suggesting a crucial role for structural MRI in predicting future conversion to AD (Frisoni et al., 2010; Jack et al., 2010).

Our recently introduced *BrainAGE* approach (Franke et al., 2010, 2012b) takes into account the widespread but sequential age-related brain tissue loss. Based on single time-point structural MRI the complex, multidimensional aging patterns across the whole brain are aggregated to one single value, i.e. the estimated brain age (Figure 1.4A; page 21). Consequently, although using only a standard MRI scan, the deviation in brain atrophy from normal brain aging can be directly quantified (Figure 1.4B; page 21). We already demonstrated that the *BrainAGE* approach is capable of identifying pathological brain aging in subjects with MCI and AD, and observed profound relationships between *BrainAGE*, disease severity and prospective worsening of cognitive functions (Franke et al., 2012a).

In order to explore the potential of applying the *BrainAGE* approach in early detection of abnormal brain changes, this study implemented this novel MRI-based biomarker to predict the conversion from MCI to AD within a time span of 36 months. We hypothesized that those individuals with greater *BrainAGE* scores would convert to AD with worse outcomes related to cognition and disease severity. Furthermore, a subsample of subjects with MCI, for whom CSF data are available, will be used to compare the performance of the *BrainAGE* framework in predicting conversion from MCI to AD to commonly used MRI and CSF biomarkers, which are widely used as state-of-the-art benchmark.

5.3 Methods
5.3.1 Subjects

We utilized data obtained from the ADNI database[25], including all MCI subjects for whom baseline MRI data (1.5T), at least moderately confident diagnoses (i.e. confidence > 2), hippocampus volumes (i.e. volumes of left and right hippocampus, calculated by FreeSurfer Version 4.3.), and test scores in certain cognitive scales (i.e. ADAS: Alzheimer's Disease Assessment Scale, range 0 – 85; CDR-SB: Clinical Dementia Rating 'sum of boxes', range 0 – 18; MMSE: Mini-Mental State Examination, range 0 – 30) were available (data downloaded in May 2010). For the exact procedures of data collection and up-to-date information, see www.adni-info.org.

Adopting the diagnostic classification at baseline and follow-up, 195 subjects were grouped as (i) *sMCI* (stable MCI), if diagnosis was MCI at all available time points, but at least for 36 months (n = 62); (ii) *pMCI_early* (progressive MCI), if diagnosis was MCI at baseline but converted to AD within the first 12 months, without reversion to MCI or cognitive normal (NO) at any available follow-up (n = 58); (iii) *pMCI_late*, if diagnosis was MCI at baseline and con-

---
[25] www.loni.ucla.edu/ADNI

version to AD was reported after the first 12 months (i.e., at 18, 24, or 36 months follow-up), without reversion to MCI or NO at any available follow-up (n = 75). Details of the characteristics of the ADNI test sample are presented in Table 5.1.

To compare the performance of the *BrainAGE* framework in predicting conversion from MCI to AD to the commonly used CSF biomarkers Aβ_{42}, total and phosphorylated tau (T-Tau and P-Tau), a subsample of subjects with MCI, for whom those CSF data are available, is utilized (Table 5.1). Adopting the same criteria as described above, this subsample is grouped as $sMCI^{CSF}$ (n = 33), $pMCI^{CSF}\_early$ (n = 32), and $pMCI^{CSF}\_late$ (n = 34). In terms of the main baseline characteristics (i.e., age, gender, education, cognition, hippocampus volumes), the CSF subsample was representative of the whole MCI sample used in this study (see Table 5.1).

To train and test the age estimation framework with respect to prediction accuracy and reliability, we used MRI data of healthy subjects from the publicly accessible IXI cohort[26] (data downloaded in February 2009) aged 50 years and older. To evaluate the accuracy of the age estimations, the subjects were divided into training and evaluation samples, i.e. after sorting the subjects by age every fourth subject entered the evaluation sample. Since the number of training samples was found to have the strongest influence on the accuracy of age prediction, MRI data of healthy subjects from the publicly accessible database OASIS[27] (data downloaded in June 2009) aged 50 years and older were also included in the training sample. In sum the training sample includes 320 cognitive normal elderly subjects. Details of the characteristics of the training sample are presented in Table 5.2.

---

[26] www.brain-development.org
[27] www.oasis-brains.org

Table 5.1: Baseline characteristics of the MCI samples used in this study.

	Whole sample (n = 195)			
	pMCI_early	pMCI_late	sMCI	F statistic (group)
No. subjects	58	75	62	–
Males / Females	33 / 25	48 / 27	49 / 13	–
Age range	55 – 86	56 – 88	58 – 88	–
Age (SD)	73.9 (7.0)	75.2 (7.3)	76.4 (6.2)	1.85 [p = 0.16]
Educational years (SD)	15.4 (2.9)	16.0 (2.9)	16.5 (2.6)	2.24 [p = 0.11]
MMSE score (SD)	26.5 (1.9)	26.8 (1.6)	27.7 (1.8)	**8.67** [**p < 0.001**]
CDR-SB score (SD)	2.0 (0.9)	1.8 (1.0)	1.3 (0.7)	**8.97** [**p < 0.001**]
ADAS score (SD)	23.5 (6.3)	20.4 (4.3)	16.3 (5.8)	**26.60** [**p < 0.001**]
Left hippocampus volume (SD)	2909 (473)	2923 (551)	3261 (479)	**9.75** [**p < 0.001**]
Right hippocampus volume (SD)	2950 (506)	2963 (551)	3276 (476)	**8.07** [**p < 0.001**]
T-Tau (SD)	–	–	–	–
P-Tau (SD)	–	–	–	–
$A\beta_{42}$ (SD)	–	–	–	–

[*Notes:* **Bold** type = significant test results.]

5.3.2 Preprocessing of MRI data and data reduction

Preprocessing of the T1-weighted images was done using the SPM8 package[28] and the VBM8 toolbox[29], running under MATLAB. All T1-weighted images were corrected for bias-field inhomogeneities, then spatially normalized and segmented into grey matter, white matter, and CSF within the same generative model (Ashburner and Friston, 2005). The segmentation procedure

---

[28] www.fil.ion.ucl.ac.uk/spm
[29] http://dbm.neuro.uni-jena.de

Table 5.1 (continued): Baseline characteristics of the MCI samples used in this study.

	CSF subsample (n = 99)			F statistic (group)	F statistic (group x subsample)
	pMCI^{CSF}_early	pMCI^{CSF}_late	sMCI^{CSF}		
No. subjects	32	34	33	–	–
Males / Females	18 / 14	13 / 11	27 / 6	–	–
Age range	55 – 86	58 – 88	63 – 88	–	–
Age (SD)	73.4 (7.0)	76.3 (7.7)	76.3 (5.8)	1.88 [$p = 0.16$]	0.83 [$p = 0.44$]
Educational years (SD)	15.2 (3.1)	15.7 (3.0)	16.6 (2.4)	1.84 [$p = 0.16$]	0.29 [$p = 0.75$]
MMSE score (SD)	26.4 (2.0)	26.6 (1.6)	27.4 (1.8)	2.58 [$p = 0.08$]	0.46 [$p = 0.63$]
CDR-SB score (SD)	2.0 (0.9)	1.7 (1.1)	1.3 (0.6)	4.23 [$p < 0.05$]	0.07 [$p = 0.93$]
ADAS score (SD)	22.9 (5.7)	20.3 (4.4)	16.5 (6.3)	10.72 [$p < 0.001$]	0.45 [$p = 0.63$]
Left hippocampus volume (SD)	2821 (482)	2907 (516)	3273 (447)	8.09 [$p < 0.001$]	0.76 [$p = 0.47$]
Right hippocampus volume (SD)	2873 (447)	2878 (529)	3255 (436)	7.07 [$p < 0.01$]	0.29 [$p = 0.75$]
T-Tau (SD)	113.8 (54.6)	116.8 (46.6)	99.2 (54.1)	1.11 [$p = 0.33$]	–
P-Tau (SD)	44.7 (17.1)	39.2 (15.6)	34.9 (18.0)	2.77 [$p = 0.07$]	–
Aβ_{42} (SD)	142.5 (35.7)	147.3 (38.2)	168.5 (62.9)	2.77 [$p = 0.07$]	–

was further extended by accounting for partial volume effects (Tohka et al., 2004), by applying adaptive maximum a posteriori estimations (Rajapakse et al., 1997), and by using a hidden Markov random field model (Cuadra et al., 2005) as described previously (Gaser, 2009). Only grey matter (GM) images were used. Following the pipeline proposed by Franke et al. (2010), the images were processed with affine registration and smoothed with 8 mm full-width-at-half-maximum (FWHM) smoothing kernels. After smoothing, spatial resolution was set to 8 mm. Then, data reduction was performed by applying principal component analysis (PCA), utilizing the "MATLAB Toolbox for Dimen-

Table 5.2: Characteristics of the samples used to model normal brain aging.

	Training sample (n = 320)		Evaluation sample
	IXI	OASIS	(IXI)
No. subjects	194	126	64
Males / Females	72 / 122	35 / 91	24 / 40
Age mean (SD)	63.5 (7.6)	71.3 (11.8)	63.5 (7.5)
Age range	51 – 86	51 – 94	51 – 83

sionality Reduction"[30]. PCA was only performed on the training sample and the estimated transformation parameters were subsequently applied to the test sample. No further data reduction or region pre-selection was accomplished.

5.3.3 Relevance vector regression (RVR)

Relevance vector machines (RVM) were introduced by Tipping (2000) as a Bayesian alternative to support vector machines (SVM) for obtaining sparse solutions to pattern recognition tasks. The main idea behind SVMs is the transformation of training data from input space into high-dimensional space – the feature space – via a mapping function Φ (Bennett and Campbell, 2003; Schölkopf and Smola, 2002). For the purpose of classification, the hyperplane that best separates the groups is computed within this feature space, resulting in a nonlinear decision boundary within the input space. The best-separating hyperplane is found by maximizing the margin between the two groups. The data points lying on the margin boundaries are called support plane. For the case of real-valued output functions (rather than just binary outputs as used in classification), the SV algorithm was generalized to regression estimation (Bennett and Campbell, 2003; Schölkopf and Smola, 2002). In support vector regression (SVR), a function has to be found that fits as many data points as possible. Analogous to the margin in classification,

---

[30] http://ict.ewi.tudelft.nl/~lvandermaaten/Home.html

the regression line is surrounded by a tube. Data points lying within that tube do not influence the course of the regression line. Data points lying on the edge or outside that tube are called support vectors.

In contrast to the support vectors in SVM, the relevance vectors in RVM represent the prototypical examples within the specified classification or regression task, instead of solely representing separating attributes. Furthermore, severe overfitting associated with the maximum likelihood estimation of the model parameters was avoided by imposing an explicit zero-mean Gaussian prior (Ghosh and Mujumdar, 2008; Zheng et al., 2008). This prior is a characteristic feature of the RVM, and its use results in a vector of independent hyperparameters that reduces the data set (Faul and Tipping, 2002; Tipping, 2000; Tipping and Faul, 2003). Therefore, in most cases the number of relevance vectors is much smaller than the number of support vectors. Furthermore, in SVR additional parameters have to be determined or statistically optimized (e.g. with cross-validation loops) in order to control for model complexity and model fit. To control the behavior of the RVR, only the type of kernel has to be chosen, whereas all other parameters are automatically estimated by the learning procedure itself. More details can be found in Bishop (2006), Schölkopf and Smola (2002), and Tipping (2000).

5.3.4 Age estimation framework

The *BrainAGE* framework utilizes RVR (Tipping, 2001) and was recently developed to estimate individual brain ages based on T1-weighted images (Franke et al., 2010). As suggested by Franke et al. (2010), the kernel was chosen to be a polynomial of degree 1, since age estimation accuracy was shown to not improve when choosing non-linear kernels. Thus, parameter optimization during the training procedure was not necessary.

In general, the model is trained with preprocessed whole brain structural MRI data (as described in section 5.3.2) of the training sample. Subsequently, the brain age of a test subject can be estimated using the individual tissue-classified MRI data, aggregating the complex, multi-dimensional aging pattern across the whole brain into one single value. The difference between estimated and true chronological age will reveal the individual *"Brain Age Gap Estimation"* (*BrainAGE*) score. Consequently, the *BrainAGE* score directly quantifies the amount of acceleration or deceleration of brain aging. For example, if a 70 years old individual has a *BrainAGE* score of +5 years, this means that this individual shows the typical atrophy pattern of a 75 years old individual. For training the model as well as for predicting individual brain ages, we used "The Spider"[31], a freely available toolbox running under MATLAB. More detailed information as well as the most important features data that were used by the RVR for estimating the brain age can be found in Franke et al. (2010).

Within this study, the framework was separately trained on male and female subjects in the training sample. With a mean absolute error of 3.8 years in the evaluation sample of healthy subjects the framework showed accurate performance in brain age estimation. Subsequently, the brain ages of the test subjects were estimated based on their baseline MRI data. The difference between the estimated and the true age resulted in the *BrainAGE* score, indicating accelerated (positive values) or decelerated (negative values) brain aging. PCA was performed on the training sample and the estimated transformation parameters were subsequently applied to the test subjects.

5.3.5 Statistical analysis

The baseline *BrainAGE* scores as well as the cognitive scores (i.e. MMSE, CDR-SB, ADAS), the hippocampus volumes, and the CSF biomarker levels at baseline were compared between the diagnostic groups in both MCI test samples using an analysis of variance (ANOVA). To assess the relationship

---

[31] www.kyb.mpg.de/bs/people/spider/main.html

between *BrainAGE* and cognitive measures at baseline and follow-up, Pearson's pairwise correlation was computed.

Receiver operating characteristics (ROC) for discriminating MCI subjects who converted to AD from those who remained stable during follow-up were computed in both MCI samples, resulting in the area under the ROC curve (AUC), which is also known as C-statistics or c-index. The AUC shows the quality of the classification, with 1.0 indicating a perfect discrimination and 0.5 indicating a result obtained by chance only. In order to test whether the resulting AUC derived from ROC analysis with *BrainAGE* is statistically greater than the AUCs of cognitive scores, hippocampus volumes, and CSF biomarkers, one-tailed z-tests are performed. Additionally, the McNemar test for paired data was performed in order to statistically test whether predictions of conversion based on baseline *BrainAGE* scores are significantly better than predictions based on cognitive scores, hippocampus volumes, and CSF biomarkers.

Likelihood ratios were computed to determine the likelihood that a *BrainAGE* score or biomarker value above a determined threshold would be expected in pMCI relative to sMCI subjects. These ratios determined whether the use of a clinical biomarker substantially changes the post-test probability that a subject will convert to AD.

Within both MCI samples, univariate Cox regression was used to estimate the hazard rate for conversion to AD, adjusting for age, education years, and gender. The time-to-event variable was time from baseline visit to first visit with AD diagnosis for pMCI subjects. For sMCI subjects, the duration of follow-up was truncated at 3 years. The main predictor was the baseline *BrainAGE* score as a continuous variable initially and in quartiles subsequently. For comparison, Cox regression was also performed with baseline cognitive scores, hippocampus volumes, and CSF biomarkers as main predictors. As checked by log-minus-log-plots of survival, the assumption of proportional hazards was met for all Cox proportional hazard models. Cox regression was performed using SPSS. All other statistical testing was performed using MATLAB.

5.4 Results
5.4.1 Whole MCI sample

The diagnostic groups (i.e. pMCI_early, pMCI_late, sMCI) did not differ in terms age and education years (Table 5.1). As expected, at baseline examination all cognitive scores as well as the hippocampus volumes differed between groups (Figure 5.1B-F).

The baseline *BrainAGE* scores significantly differed between the diagnostic groups ($F = 26.04$, $p < 0.001$), resulting in the following means: pMCI_early = 8.73 years, pMCI_late = 5.62 years, and sMCI = 0.75 years. As mentioned above, positive values indicate a higher estimated than chronological age. Post hoc t-tests showed significant differences ($p < 0.05$) between all three diagnostic groups (Figure 5.1A).

As expected, cognitive abilities substantially declined during the follow-up intervals in both pMCI groups but remained stable in those who did not convert to AD (Figure 5.2A-C). Statistically significant correlations at baseline were only found between *BrainAGE* scores and CDR-SB as well as ADAS, but not for MMSE (Table 5.3). During follow-up, the correlations between baseline *BrainAGE* scores and clinical disease severity as well as cognitive functioning even increased, denoting a close relationship between pathological brain aging and prospective worsening of cognitive functioning.

Our test sample included 195 subjects diagnosed with MCI at baseline. During 36 months of follow-up, a total of 133 of them developed AD, corresponding to a pre-test probability of 68%. More specifically, 30% of the MCI subjects converted to AD within the first 12 months after baseline examina-

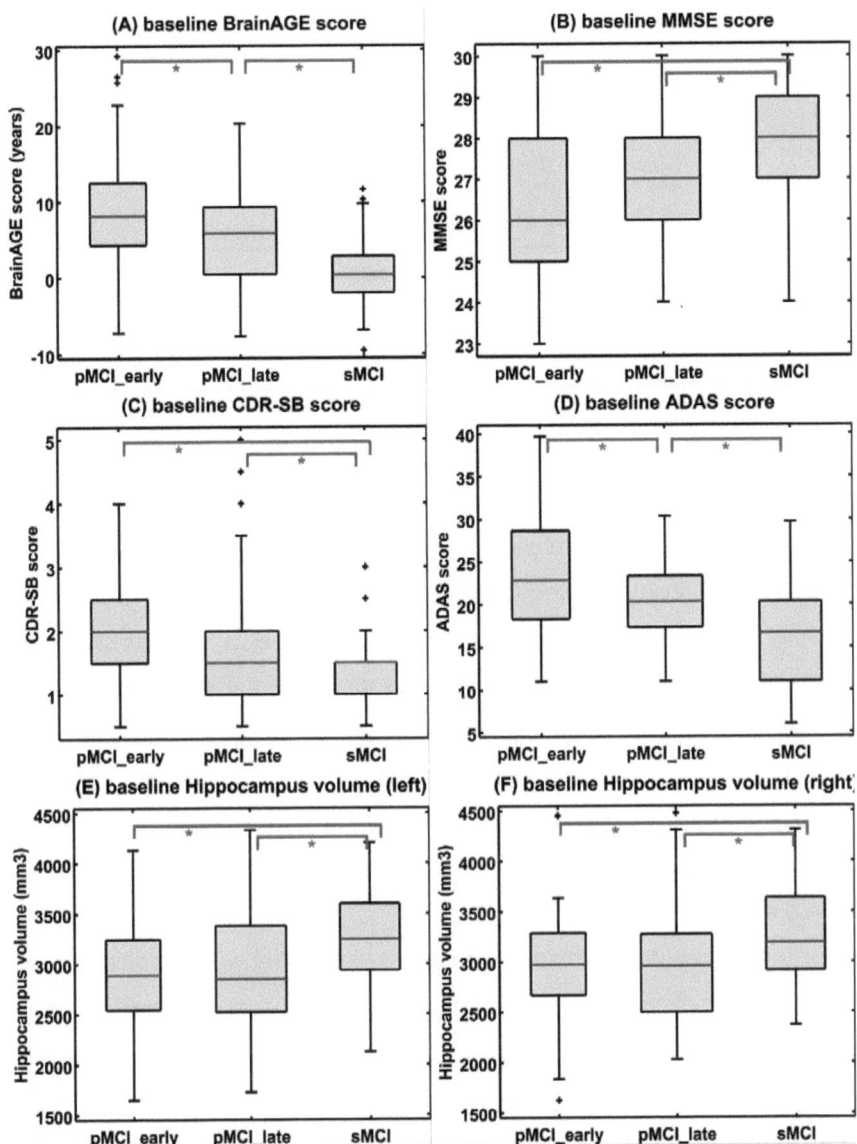

Figure 5.1: Baseline scores in all MCI groups. Shown are box plots for baseline **(A)** *BrainAGE* scores (in years), **(B)** MMSE scores, **(C)** CDR-SB scores, **(D)** ADAS scores, **(E)** left and **(F)** right hippocampus volumes (in mm^3) of all diagnostic groups. Post-hoc t- tests resulting in significant differences between diagnostic groups are indicated ($p < 0.05$; red lines). The boxes contain the values between the 25th and 75th percentiles, including the median (gray line). Lines extending above and below each box symbolize data within 1.5 times the interquartile range (outliers are displayed with a +). Width of the boxes indicates the group size. [Figure and legend modified from Gaser et al. 2013.]

Table 5.3: Results for correlation analyses of baseline *BrainAGE* scores with cognitive scores at baseline and follow-up (whole sample).

	baseline	6 months follow-up	12 months follow-up	18 months follow-up	24 months follow-up	36 months follow-up
MMSE	−0.09	−0.17*	−0.25***	−0.24**	−0.39***	−0.41***
CDR-SB	0.20**	0.26***	0.28***	0.32***	0.42***	0.46***
ADAS	0.23**	0.24**	0.35***	0.38***	0.44***	0.48***

[*Notes:* *p < 0.05, **p < 0.01, ***p < 0.001.]

tion (mean time to conversion: 312 ± 96 days), whereas 38% of all MCI subjects converted to AD after the first year of follow-up (mean time to conversion: 705 ± 228 days). By varying the threshold applied to the *BrainAGE* score, we constructed ROC curves for a binary discrimination between MCI subjects who remained stable during 3 years follow-up from those who converted to AD. With AUCs (or c-index) of 0.83 and 0.78, and accuracy rates of 81% and 75% for the discrimination of sMCI vs. pMCI_early (Figure 5.3A) and all pMCI subjects (Figure 5.3B), respectively, the baseline *BrainAGE* score proved its encouraging potential to predict conversion to AD in MCI subjects. Furthermore, predicting future conversion to AD based on baseline *BrainAGE* scores was significantly more accurate than predictions based on chronological age, hippocampus volumes, and cognitive scores at baseline (Table 5.4).

For the whole MCI sample the post-test probability was increased to 90% when using baseline *BrainAGE* scores to predict conversion to AD within 36 months of follow-up (Figure 5.4A). This gain in certainty by 22% was highest for the baseline *BrainAGE* score as compared to baseline hippocampus volumes (right hippocampus: 16%; left hippocampus: 17%) or cognitive scores (MMSE: 11%; CDR-SB: 0%; ADAS: 18%).

Cox regression analysis showed an association of higher *BrainAGE* scores with a higher risk of developing AD ($\chi^2 = 58.86$, $p < 0.001$; Table 5.5).

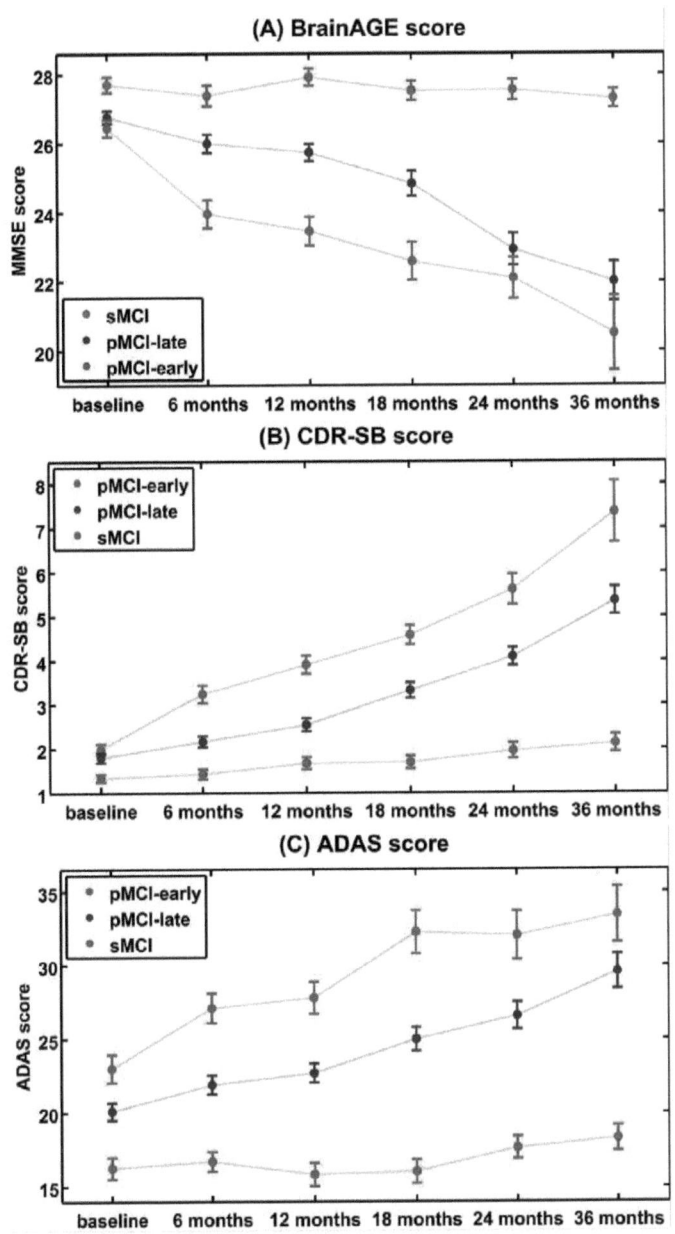

Figure 5.2: Cognitive scores during follow-up. Mean **(A)** MMSE, **(B)** CDR-SB, **(C)** ADAS scores in pMCI_early, pMCI_ate, and sMCI subjects at baseline examination as well as all follow-up assessments. Error bars depict the standard error of the mean (SEM). [Figure and legend modified from Gaser et al. 2013.]

Table 5.4: Results for predicting conversion to AD in MCI subjects with baseline scores (whole sample).

	pMCI_early				
	Accuracy [CI]	Sensitivity [CI]	Specificity [CI]	McNemar test	
				Error rate [CI]	χ^2
BrainAGE score	0.81 [0.74–0.88]	0.78 [0.70–0.85]	0.84 [0.77–0.90]	0.19 [0.12–0.26]	–
Chronological age	0.41 [0.32–0.50]	0.29 [0.21–0.37]	0.89 [0.83–0.94]	0.59 [0.50–0.68]	28.69 *[p < 0.001]*
MMSE score	0.57 [0.48–0.66]	0.71 [0.63–0.79]	0.61 [0.53–0.70]	0.43 [0.34–0.52]	13.07 *[p < 0.001]*
CDR-SB score	0.59 [0.50–0.68]	0.64 [0.55–0.72]	0.77 [0.70–0.85]	0.41 [0.32–0.50]	15.87 *[p < 0.001]*
ADAS score	0.66 [0.57–0.74]	0.65 [0.56–0.73]	0.81 [0.74–0.88]	0.34 [0.26–0.43]	5.90 *[p < 0.05]*
Left hippocampus volume	0.66 [0.57–0.74]	0.52 [0.43–0.61]	0.81 [0.74–0.88]	0.34 [0.26–0.43]	6.42 *[p < 0.05]*
Right hippocampus volume	0.61 [0.52–0.70]	0.84 [0.78–0.91]	0.42 [0.33–0.51]	0.39 [0.30–0.48]	9.62 *[p < 0.01]*

Each additional year in the *BrainAGE* score was associated with a 10% greater risk of developing AD (hazard rate: 1.10, $p < 0.001$; Table 5.5). Compared with subjects in the lowest *BrainAGE* quartile (−9.55 – −0.12 years), subjects in the 2nd quartile (−0.12 – 4.45 years) had about the same risk of developing AD (hazard ratio [HR]: 1.13 [95% confidence interval (CI): 0.62 – 2.06], $p = 0.68$), those in the 3rd quartile (4.46 – 9.26 years) had a three times greater risk (HR: 3.12 [CI: 1.80 – 5.40], $p < 0.001$), and those in the 4th quartile (9.26 – 29.20 years) had a four times greater risk (HR: 4.66 [CI: 2.61 – 8.29], $p < 0.001$) of developing AD (Figure 5.5). Thus, MCI subjects showing abnormal atrophy patterns as marked by higher *BrainAGE* scores had a significantly increased risk and a cumulative probability of 88% in the 3rd quartile and 92% in the 4th quartile for conversion to AD. Furthermore, when performing Cox regression with all other baseline scores, *BrainAGE* again showed the best results (Table 5.5, Figure 5.6).

Table 5.4 *(continued)*: Results for predicting conversion to AD in MCI subjects with baseline scores (whole sample).

	pMCI (all)				
	Accuracy [CI]	Sensitivity [CI]	Specificity [CI]	McNemar test	
				Error rate [CI]	χ^2
BrainAGE score	0.75 [0.69–0.81]	0.71 [0.65–0.78]	0.84 [0.79–0.89]	0.25 [0.19–0.31]	–
Chronological age	0.52 [0.45–0.59]	0.31 [0.24–0.37]	0.85 [0.80–0.90]	0.48 [0.41–0.55]	15.87 [p < 0.001]
MMSE score	0.37 [0.31–0.44]	0.71 [0.64–0.77]	0.61 [0.54–0.68]	0.63 [0.56–0.69]	50.75 [p < 0.001]
CDR-SB score	0.38 [0.31–0.45]	0.52 [0.45–0.59]	0.77 [0.72–0.83]	0.62 [0.55–0.69]	56.47 [p < 0.001]
ADAS score	0.48 [0.41–0.55]	0.89 [0.84–0.93]	0.48 [0.41–0.55]	0.52 [0.45–0.59]	31.02 [p < 0.001]
Left hippocampus volume	0.61 [0.54–0.68]	0.53 [0.46–0.60]	0.81 [0.75–0.86]	0.39 [0.32–0.46]	8.19 [p < 0.01]
Right hippocampus volume	0.54 [0.47–0.61]	0.43 [0.36–0.50]	0.84 [0.79–0.89]	0.46 [0.39–0.53]	16.00 [p < 0.001]

5.4.2 MCI subsample with CSF data

When comparing *BrainAGE* to state-of-the-art CSF biomarkers within this multicenter study, only the baseline *BrainAGE* scores significantly differed between the diagnostic groups in the CSF subsample (sMCI^{CSF}: 0.71 years; pMCI^{CSF}_late: 5.04; pMCI^{CSF}_early: 8.20; $F = 10.82$, $p < 0.001$; Figure 5.7), but none of the baseline CSF biomarker levels (Table 5.1). *BrainAGE* scores in the CSF subsample did not differ between from those in the whole MCI sample ($F = 0.15$, $p = 0.86$).

ROC analyses with baseline *BrainAGE* scores resulted in AUCs (or c-index) of 0.84 and 0.75, and accuracy rates accuracy rates of 80% and 72% for the discrimination of sMCI^{CSF} vs. pMCI^{CSF} in early converters (Figure 5.8A) and in the whole CSF subsample (Figure 5.8B), respectively. Thus, baseline *BrainAGE* scores showed significantly better predictions than baseline T-Tau, P-Tau, and Aβ_{42} levels (Table 5.6).

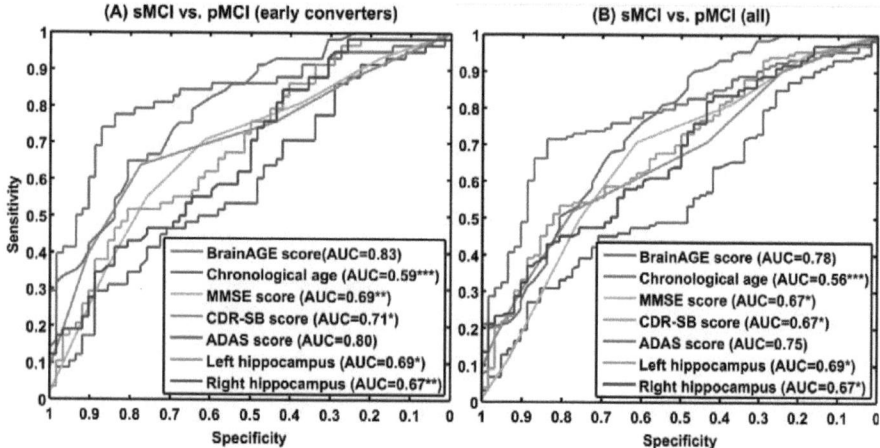

Figure 5.3: ROC curves of individual subject classification to sMCI or pMCI. ROC curves of individual subject classification to sMCI or pMCI based on baseline *BrainAGE* scores, cognitive scores, and hippocampus volumes for **(A)** early converters and **(B)** the whole sample. The areas under the ROC curves (AUCs) of cognitive scores and hippocampus volumes were tested against the AUC of *BrainAGE*. [Notes: * $p < 0.05$, ** $p < 0.01$, *** $p < 0.001$. Figure and legend modified from Gaser et al. 2013.]

Furthermore, when looking at the post-test probability in the CSF subsample, the pre-test probability of 67% for converting to AD within three years was increased by 21% using baseline *BrainAGE* scores (Figure 5.4B), but only slightly by using CSF biomarkers (T-Tau: 4%, P-Tau: 0%, Aβ_{42}: 0%, Aβ_{42}/P-Tau: 8%).

Also in the CSF subsample, Cox regression analysis showed a significant association of higher *BrainAGE* scores with a higher risk of developing AD ($\chi^2 = 22.11$, $p < 0.001$; Table 5.5). In contrast, Cox regression with CSF biomarkers did not yield significant results for any of them (Table 5.7, Figure 5.9).

5.5 Discussion

The scope of this study was the implementation of a novel MRI-based biomarker based on the recently presented *BrainAGE* framework (Franke et

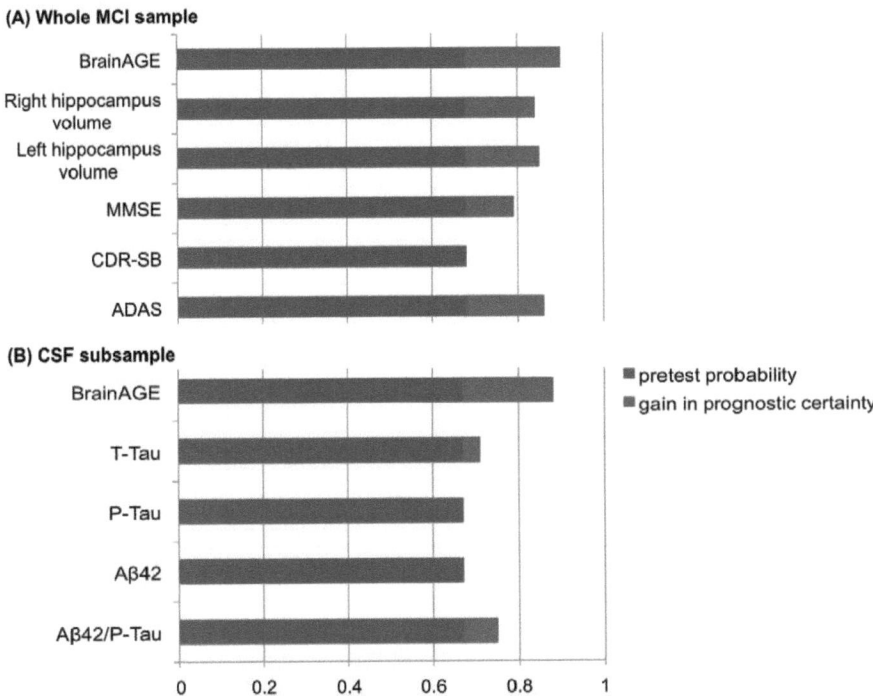

Figure 5.4: Pre-test and post-test probability for predicting conversion to AD. Pre-test probability (blue) and post-test probability (blue + red), indicating the gain in prognostic certainty (red) for predicting conversion to AD within 36 months, based on **(A)** baseline *BrainAGE* scores, hippocampus volume, and cognitive measures within the whole MCI sample, as well as **(B)** baseline *BrainAGE* scores and CSF biomarkers in the CSF subsample. [Figure and legend from Gaser et al. 2013.]

al., 2010) to predict prospective cognitive decline and conversion to AD on an individual subject level. Using structural MRI data, our fully automated age estimation model aggregates the complex, multidimensional aging patterns across the whole brain to one single value (i.e. the *BrainAGE* score) and finally identifies pathological brain aging in MCI subjects who finally converted to AD within three years of follow-up, with increasing *BrainAGE* scores at baseline indicating an increased risk of developing AD.

Table 5.5: Model statistics of Cox regression for all baseline scores (adjusted for age, gender, and education).

	Continuous predictors				
	Overall model		Continuous values		
	χ^2	p	Hazard rate [CI]	Wald statistics	p
BrainAGE score (+)	58.86	***	1.10 [1.07–1.13]	45.05	***
MMSE score (−)	28.99	***	0.81 [0.73–0.90]	16.01	***
CDR-SB score (+)	30.46	***	1.15 [1.26–1.82]	19.41	***
ADAS score (+)	56.02	***	1.11 [1.07–1.14]	40.48	***
Left hippocampus volume (−)	34.54	***	1.00 [1.00–1.00]	21.82	***
Right hippocampus volume (−)	31.65	***	1.00 [1.00–1.00]	18.90	***

[*Notes:* (+) = higher values mean higher risk for AD, (−) = lower values mean higher risk for AD.

This method already showed the advantage of accurately and reliably estimating the age of the brain with minimal preprocessing and parameter optimization (Franke et al., 2010, 2012b), using a single anatomical scan. Regarding the relevance within the clinical context, higher *BrainAGE* scores were recently demonstrated to be closely related to measures of clinical disease severity in AD patients, as well as prospective worsening of cognitive functioning in MCI subjects who converted to AD within three years (Franke et al., 2012a). Furthermore, already possessing higher *BrainAGE* scores at baseline, brain atrophy was shown to even accelerate during follow-up, with the speed of one additional year per follow-up year in pMCI subjects and 1.5 additional years per follow-up year in AD patients. Considering unequal follow-up durations in the pMCI and AD groups, this finally accumulated to mean *BrainAGE* scores of about 9 years at the last scan in both groups. Compared to that, sMCI and healthy control subjects did not show any irregularity in brain atrophy at baseline and follow-up (Franke et al., 2012a).

Table 5.5 *(continued)*: Model statistics of Cox regression for all baseline scores (adjusted for age, gender, and education).

	Categorical predictors (median split)			
	Overall model		Values below vs. above median		
	χ^2	p	Hazard ratio [CI]	Wald statistics	p
BrainAGE score (+)	**52.23**	*******	**3.41 [2.30–5.07]**	**37.03**	*******
MMSE score (-)	25.04	***	2.02 [1.37–2.99]	12.55	***
CDR-SB score (+)	26.74	***	1.97 [1.38–2.82]	13.89	***
ADAS score (+)	29.78	***	2.12 [1.48–3.03]	16.84	***
Left hippocampus volume (-)	23.84	***	1.91 [1.31–2.78]	11.34	**
Right hippocampus volume (-)	18.56	**	1.59 [1.11–2.28]	6.32	*

[* $p < 0.05$, ** $p < 0.01$, *** $p < 0.001$. **Bold** type = best performance of all markers.]

In the study presented here, the *BrainAGE* approach was implemented to predict subsequent conversion to AD on a single subject level based on structural MRI at baseline. Focusing on subjects with mild memory impairment but preserved activities of daily life, we found accuracy rates of up to 81% for prediction of progression to AD. Even more interestingly, a high *BrainAGE* score increased the prognostic certainty of a subsequent conversion to AD from 68% in our clinically defined MCI sample to 90%. This gain in certainty may provide solid diagnostic grounds for early intervention strategies aimed at delaying or preventing the onset of full-scale AD in subjects at highest risk for the disease. Furthermore, our *BrainAGE* framework was more precise in predicting conversion of MCI to AD when compared to chronological age, cognitive scores, hippocampus volume, or state-of-the-art CSF biomarkers.

Cognitive decline was recently found to progressively accelerate years before being diagnosed as AD (Wilson et al., 2011), and to be correlated with

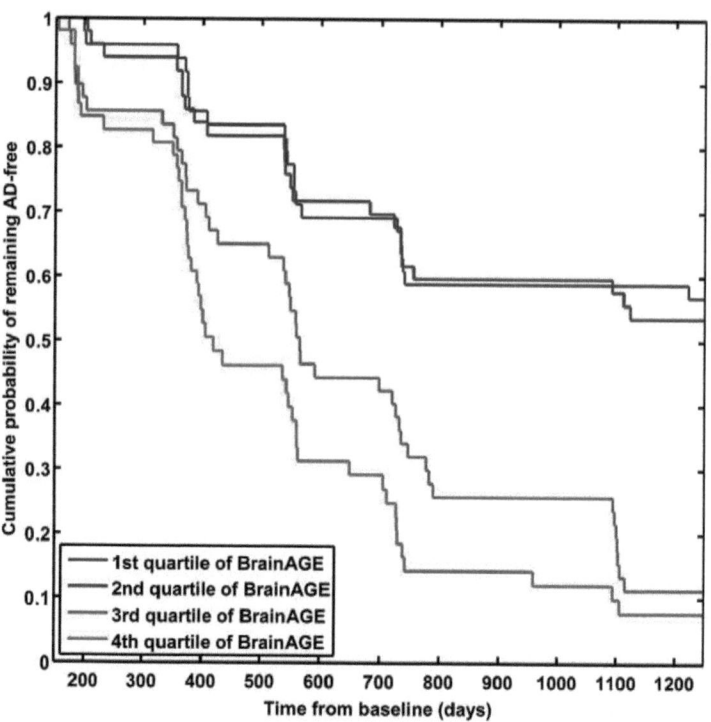

Figure 5.5: Cumulative probability of remaining AD-free in the quartiles of baseline *BrainAGE* score. Kaplan-Meier survival curves based on Cox regression comparing cumulative AD incidence in subjects with MCI at baseline by *BrainAGE* score quartiles (p for trend < 0.001). Duration of follow-up is truncated at 1250 days. [Figure and legend from Gaser et al. 2013.]

the atrophy rates in specified brain regions (Desikan et al., 2008). In addition, some studies focusing on regression methods to identify pathological brain structures specific for AD reported moderate performance measures when predicting one-year decline of cognitive functions in MCI (Duchesne et al., 2009; Stonnington et al., 2010; Wang et al., 2010). Although not specifically trained to predict changes in cognitive scales, the *BrainAGE* scores estimated at baseline showed moderate correlations with measures of clinical disease severity and cognitive functioning up to three years in advance. These results as well as our recent results from a longitudinal *BrainAGE*

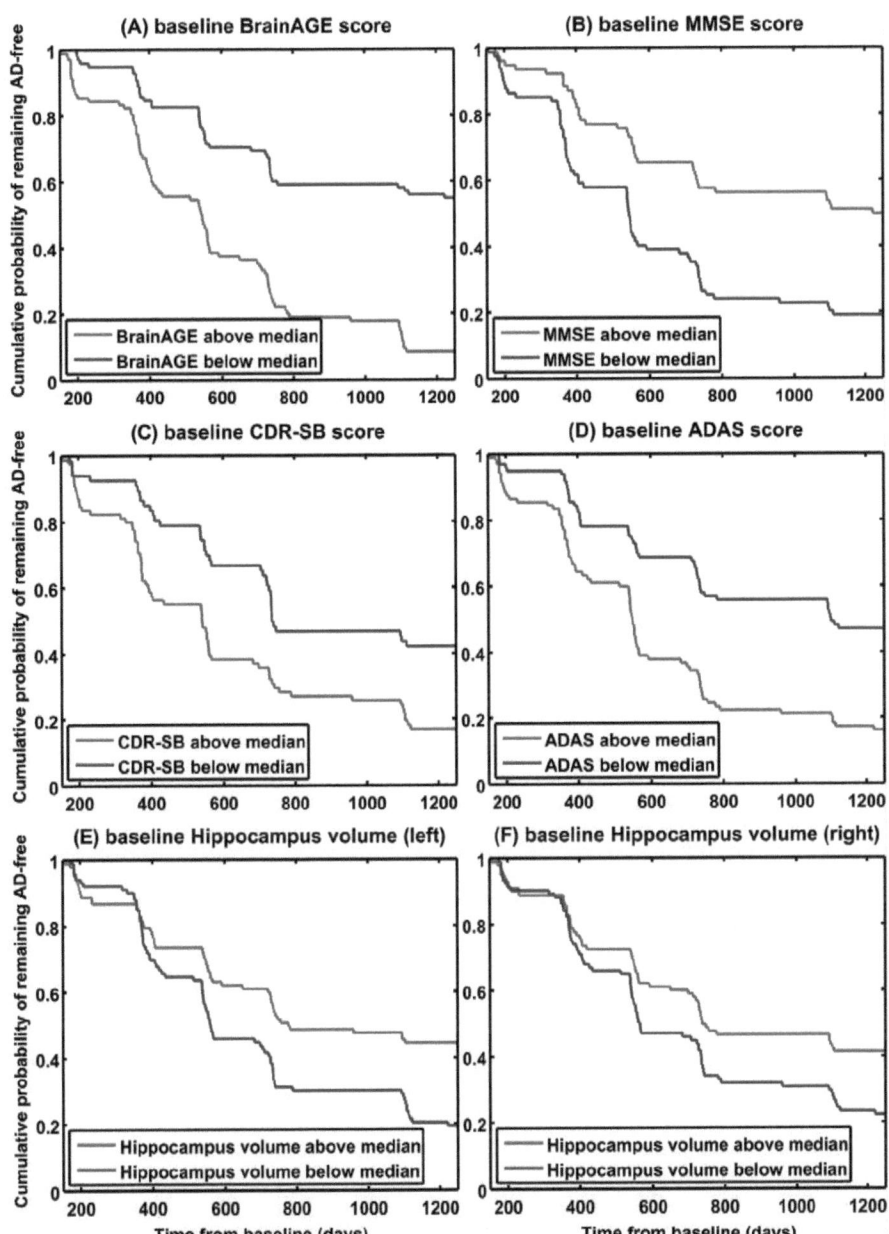

Figure 5.6: **Cumulative probability of remaining AD-free in the whole MCI sample.** Kaplan-Meier survival curves based on Cox regression comparing cumulative AD incidence in subjects with MCI at baseline by all baseline scores split at median. Duration of follow-up is truncated at 1250 days. [Figure and legend modified from Gaser et al. 2013.]

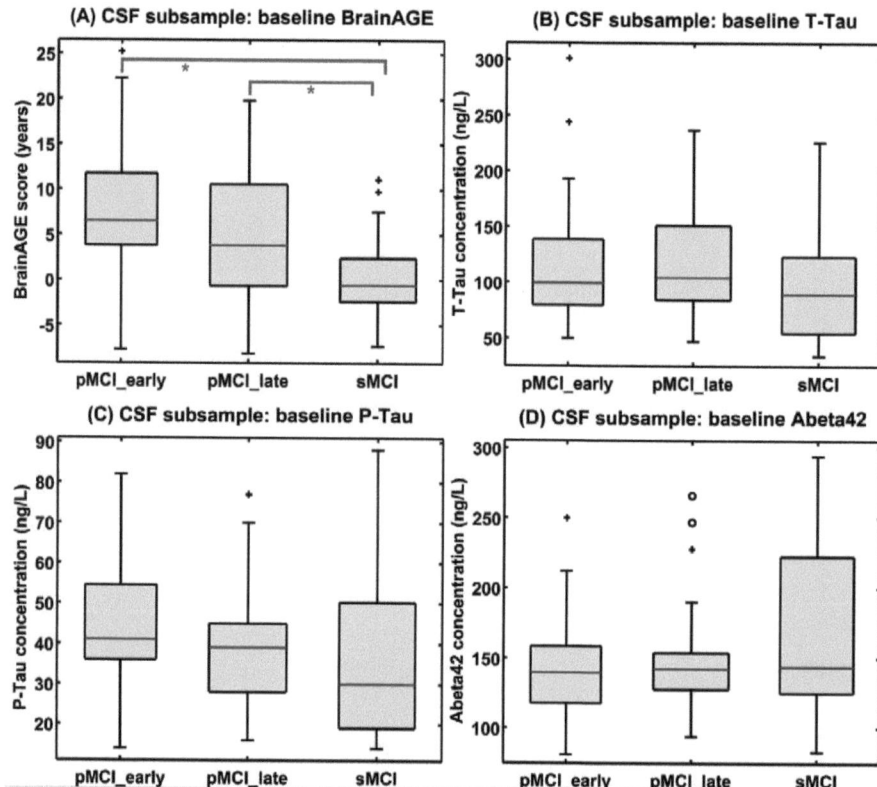

Figure 5.7: Baseline *BrainAGE* scores and baseline CSF biomarker concentrations in the MCI-subsample. Shown are box plots for **(A)** *BrainAGE* scores, **(B)** T-Tau, **(C)** P-Tau, and **(D)** $A\beta_{42}$ concentration at baseline of all diagnostic groups in the subsample that also provides CSF data. The boxes contain the values between the 25th and 75th percentiles, including the median (gray line). Lines extending above and below each box symbolize data within 1.5 times the interquartile range (outliers are displayed with a +). Width of the boxes indicates the group size. Post-hoc t-tests resulted in significant differences between diagnostic groups only for baseline *BrainAGE* scores ($p < 0.05$; red lines). [Figure and legend modified from Gaser et al. 2013.]

study (Franke et al., 2012b) support the suggested relationship between progressive acceleration in brain atrophy and worsening of cognitive functioning in progressive MCI.

Using high-dimensional pattern recognition with imaging data was recently suggested to provide a viable biomarker to detect subtle, but predictive, imaging phenotypes that precede cognitive decline while there is still opportunity

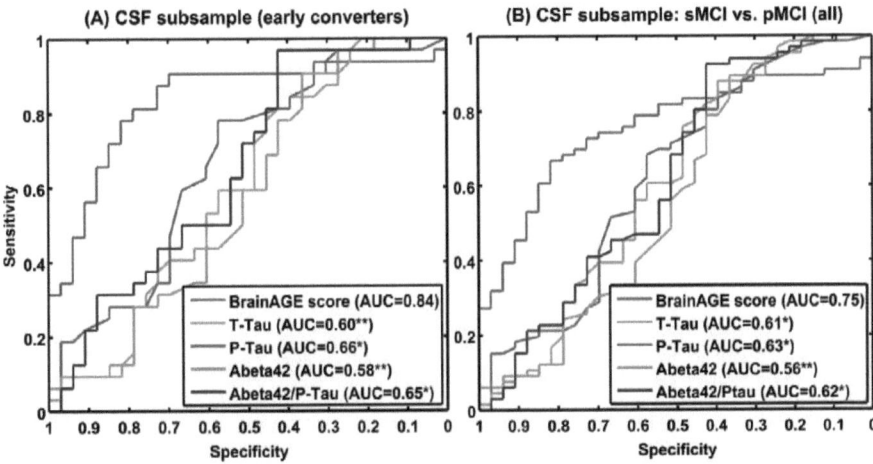

Figure 5.8: ROC curves of individual subject classification to sMCI or pMCI in the CSF subsample. ROC curves of individual subject classification to sMCI^{CSF} or pMCI^{CSF} based on baseline *BrainAGE* scores and CSF biomarkers for **(A)** early converters and **(B)** the whole CSF subsample. The areas under the ROC curves (AUCs) of the CSF biomarkers were tested against the AUC of *BrainAGE*. [Notes: * $p < 0.05$, ** $p < 0.01$. Figure and legend modified from Gaser et al. 2013.]

for preventive or therapeutic interventions (Clark et al., 2012). Current classification approaches attempt to identify disease-specific patterns that allow a separation of subjects with MCI or AD from healthy samples. Whilst most approaches are able to accurately differentiate between healthy controls and AD patients (Hinrichs et al., 2011; Walhovd et al., 2010; Zhang et al., 2011), it is the conversion from MCI to AD that is of greater clinical interest and clinical consequence. Attempting this issue, most approaches showed a substantial drop in accuracy when predicting MCI-to-AD conversion on an individual level, especially when relying on baseline data only (Davatzikos et al., 2011; Misra et al., 2009; Querbes et al., 2009; Teipel et al., 2007; Vemuri et al., 2009b; Westman et al., 2011). Nevertheless, individuals showing the first subtle signs of abnormal atrophy will benefit most from an early therapy, provided to reliably identify those individuals at risk of progressing to AD in future. For example, a recent study based on cortical thickness reported the

Table 5.6: Results in the CSF subsample for predicting conversion to AD in MCI subjects with baseline scores.

			pMCI^{CSF}_early		
	Accuracy [CI]	Sensitivity [CI]	Specificity [CI]	McNemar test Error rate [CI]	χ^2
BrainAGE score	0.80 [0.70–0.90]	0.91 [0.83–0.98]	0.70 [0.58–0.81]	0.20 [0.10–0.30]	–
T-Tau	0.60 [0.48–0.72]	0.84 [0.76–0.93]	0.39 [0.27–0.51]	0.40 [0.28–0.52]	4.80 [$p < 0.05$]
P-Tau	0.57 [0.45–0.69]	0.78 [0.68–0.88]	0.58 [0.46–0.70]	0.43 [0.31–0.55]	7.54 [$p < 0.01$]
Aβ_{42}	0.57 [0.45–0.69]	0.91 [0.83–0.98]	0.36 [0.25–0.48]	0.43 [0.31–0.55]	7.26 [$p < 0.01$]
Aβ_{42} / P-Tau	0.69 [0.58–0.80]	0.97 [0.93–1.00]	0.42 [0.30–0.54]	0.31 [0.20–0.42]	1.69 [n.s.]

[*Notes:* n.s. = not significant.]

accurate detection of 81% of those MCI subjects who were to be clinically diagnosed as AD patients 24 months later (Querbes et al., 2009). But this was only true when looking at those MCI subjects who were converting to AD, while ignoring those MCI subjects who did not convert. Consequently, the overall accuracy of sMCI vs. pMCI classification ranged from 48% at 6 months to 73% at 24 months.

Furthermore, although a very recent study reported that combining MRI and CSF measures in a multivariate model resulted in better accuracy for predicting future conversion from MCI to AD, than using either MRI or CSF separately (Westman et al., 2012), the overall prediction accuracies for converters and non-converters ranged only from 58.6% to 66.4% at different time points. With sensitivity of 67% and specificity of 69%, another recent study (Wolz et al., 2011) also achieved the most stable and reliable classification results when combining all available structural MRI features (i.e., hippocampus volume, tensor-based morphometry, cortical thickness). Thus, with accuracy rates up to 81% in predicting conversion to AD within the whole MCI

Table 5.6 (continued): Results in the CSF subsample for predicting conversion to AD in MCI subjects with baseline scores.

	pMCI^{CSF} (all)				
	Accuracy [CI]	Sensitivity [CI]	Specificity [CI]	McNemar test Error rate [CI]	χ^2
BrainAGE score	0.72 [0.63–0.81]	0.67 [0.57–0.76]	0.82 [0.74–0.89]	0.28 [0.19–0.37]	–
T-Tau	0.58 [0.48–0.76]	0.88 [0.81–0.94]	0.39 [0.30–0.49]	0.42 [0.33–0.52]	3.93 [p < 0.05]
P-Tau	0.43 [0.34–0.53]	0.68 [0.59–0.77]	0.58 [0.48–0.67]	0.57 [0.47–0.66]	16.20 [p < 0.001]
Aβ_{42}	0.49 [0.40–0.59]	0.89 [0.83–0.95]	0.36 [0.27–0.46]	0.51 [0.41–0.60]	7.08 [p < 0.01]
Aβ_{42} / P-Tau	0.73 [0.64–0.81]	0.92 [0.87–0.98]	0.42 [0.33–0.52]	0.27 [0.18–0.36]	0.03 [n.s.]

sample up to three years in advance, *BrainAGE* is comparable or even outperforms recent classification studies that predicted decline of cognitive scores in MCI subjects or short-term conversion to AD (e.g., Davatzikos et al., 2011; Fan et al., 2008a; Misra et al., 2009; Querbes et al., 2009; Teipel et al., 2007; Westman et al., 2011).

Besides and in contrast to CSF biomarkers, MRI is non-invasive and can be performed more rapidly than a detailed neuropsychological testing. Furthermore, brain imaging is part of the diagnostic work-up (Walhovd et al., 2010), with MRI becoming the imaging modality of choice in many centers. Additionally, MRI was shown to retain the closest relationship with memory loss as well as worsening of clinical functions (Jack et al., 2010). Consequently, current models of the dynamics of well established biomarkers of the Alzheimer's pathological cascade suggest a crucial role for structural MRI in predicting future cognitive decline and conversion to AD (Clark et al., 2012; Frisoni et al., 2010; Jack et al., 2010). Even though hippocampus volume has been shown to represent an independent risk factor for AD and robustly predicting conversion to AD in MCI subjects, the *BrainAGE* approach outper-

Table 5.7: Model statistics of Cox regression for all baseline scores (adjusted for age, gender, and education).

	Continuous predictors				
	Overall model		Continuous values		
	χ^2	p	Hazard rate [CI]	Wald statistics	p
BrainAGE score (+)	22.11	***	1.08 [1.04–1.12]	14.86	***
T-Tau (+)	6.90	n.s.	1.00 [1.00–1.01]	0.17	n.s.
P-Tau (+)	9.54	*	1.01 [1.00–1.03]	2.78	n.s.
Aβ_{42} (–)	10.33	*	0.99 [0.99–1.00]	3.54	n.s.
Aβ_{42} / P-Tau (–)	12.90	*	0.91 [0.84–0.98]	5.63	*

[*Notes:* (+) = higher values mean higher risk for AD, (–) = lower values mean higher risk for AD.]

formed prediction utilizing baseline hippocampus volumes in the present study as well as in recently published classification studies (Costafreda et al., 2011; Risacher et al., 2009, 2010).

One limitation of our approach might be that white matter lesions that occur primarily due to cerebro-vascular diseases are not detected in the segmentation approach. Those lesions are segmented as gray matter and might therefore influence the relevance vector regression. However, because such lesions only occur in a limited number of subjects it is very unlikely that they contribute to the relevance vectors because of their high local variance. In future, the segmentation should be extended by methods that allow an automated detection of white matter lesions even without any additional FLAIR sequence (Klöppel et al., 2011).

As stated before, the *BrainAGE* method builds on the assumption of AD being preceded by an acceleration in brain atrophy that resembles advanced aging (e.g., Cao et al., 2010; Driscoll et al., 2009; Dukart et al., 2011; Jones et al., 2011; Saetre et al., 2011; Spulber et al., 2010), although there are other studies rejecting that assumption (e.g., Nelson et al., 2011; Ohnishi et

Table 5.7 (continued): Model statistics of Cox regression for all baseline scores (adjusted for age, gender, and education).

	Overall model		Categorical predictors (median split)		
			Values below vs. above median		
	χ^2	p	Hazard ratio [CI]	Wald statistics	p
BrainAGE score (+)	**24.33**	*******	**3.41 [1.89–6.14]**	**16.75**	*******
T-Tau (+)	6.92	n.s.	1.11 [0.67–1.64]	0.15	n.s.
P-Tau (+)	7.86	n.s.	1.29 [0.77–2.14]	0.96	n.s.
$A\beta_{42}$ (-)	6.73	n.s.	0.98 [0.59–1.63]	0.00	n.s.
$A\beta_{42}$ / P-Tau (-)	6.83	n.s.	1.08 [0.66–1.78]	0.10	n.s.

* $p < 0.05$, *** $p < 0.001$, n.s. = not significant. **Bold** type = best performance of all markers.]

al., 2001). However, the acceleration of spatiotemporal brain atrophy might only be seen in subjects in a preclinical stage, while in AD patients additional disease-specific pathological changes are occurring. Further, subjects with a high BrainAGE score but no AD-specific clinical profile may suffer from other neurodegenerative diseases. This issue should be explored by applying our framework to other neurodegenerative diseases. Furthermore, cognitive reserve, genetic status, education level, socioeconomic status, lifestyle, or vitamin supply may protect subjects from pathological brain aging or accelerated cognitive decline despite high BrainAGE scores (Chen et al., 2009; Fotenos et al., 2008; Mangialasche et al., 2013; Querbes et al., 2009; Snowdon, 2003). Thus, in future research we aim to disentangle age- and unrelated disease-based processes of brain tissue loss in AD. Additionally, we will elucidate the effects of the genetic status, e.g., Apolipoprotein E (APOE), on the longitudinal changes in BrainAGE as well as on prediction of AD conversion, since especially the APOE ε4 allele is associated with modification of cognitive functioning (Cosentino et al., 2008; Deary et al., 2002; Wishart et

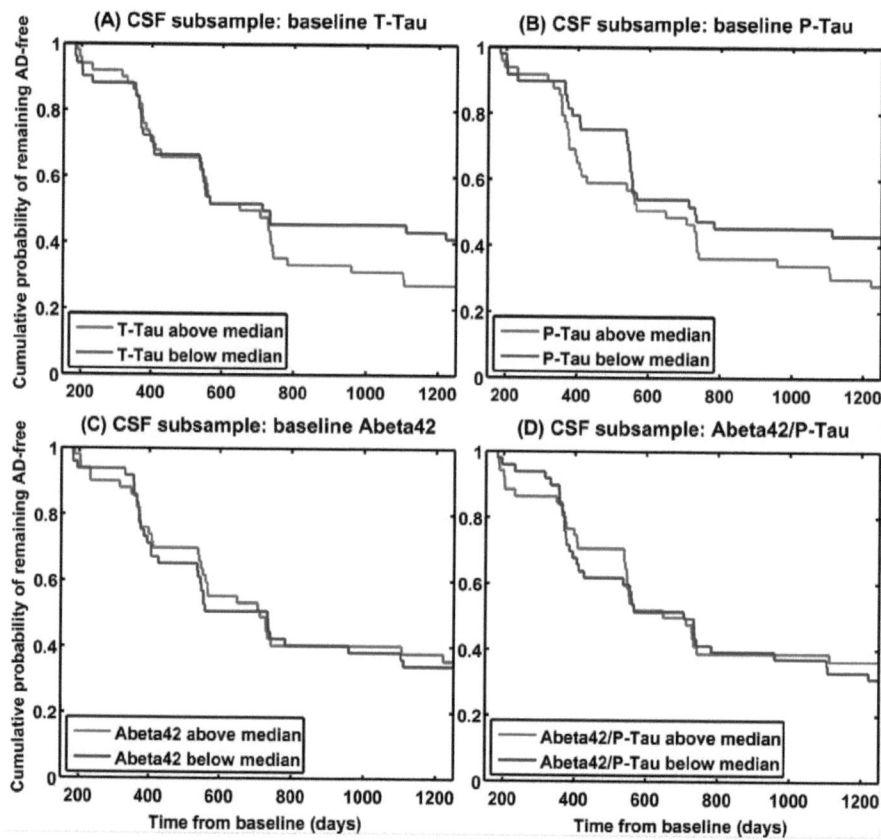

Figure 5.9: **Cumulative probability of remaining AD-free in the CSF subsample.** Kaplan-Meier survival curves based on Cox regression comparing cumulative AD incidence in subjects with MCI at baseline by all CSF biomarker baseline levels split at median. Duration of follow-up is truncated at 1250 days. [Figure and legend modified from Gaser et al. 2013.]

al., 2006) and GM reduction in AD patients (Filippini et al., 2009) as well as healthy subjects (Bookheimer et al., 2000).

In conclusion, *BrainAGE* has shown promising results on an individual level, contributing to an early indication of pathological brain aging in advance of severe clinical symptoms, or even predicting future cognitive decline. Compared to a wide range of existing classification approaches that require disease-specific data for training, the *BrainAGE* framework uses an independent database of healthy, non-demented subjects to model the normal brain-aging pattern and consequently recognizing subtle deviations from age-related brain atrophy in new test samples. As the *BrainAGE* approach utilizes only a single T1-weighted image per subject and already has proven to work fast and fully automated with multi-centre data, it can be easily implemented in clinical routine to encourage the identification of subtly abnormal atrophy patterns.[32]

---

[32] **Acknowledgments:** Data used in preparation of this article were obtained from the Alzheimer's Disease Neuroimaging Initiative (ADNI) database (http://adni.loni.ucla.edu). As such, the investigators within the ADNI contributed to the design and implementation of ADNI and / or provided data but did not participate in analysis or writing of this report. A complete listing of ADNI investigators can be found at http://adni.loni.ucla.edu/wp-content/uploads/how_to_apply/ADNI_Acknowledgement_List.pdf.

Chapter 6.
General Discussion

The general scope of this work was the development and implementation of a novel biomarker that aggregates the complex, multidimensional aging pattern across the whole brain into one single value; i.e. the *BrainAGE* score. Using structural MRI data, the *BrainAGE* score directly quantifies acceleration or deceleration in individual brain aging, thus providing clinically relevant information about normal or even abnormal age-related changes in the brain structure. In order to facilitate usability in a clinical routine, the algorithm should work fast and be fully automatic. The *BrainAGE* approach estimates the neuroanatomical brain age with minimal preprocessing and parameter optimization, using a single structural MRI scan.

6.1 Stability of *BrainAGE* estimation

The proposed *BrainAGE* approach comprises well established and fully automated processing of structural MR images to aggregate the complex, region-specific, and non-linear patterns of neurodegenerative age-related changes across the whole brain into one single value, thus providing a reference curve for healthy brain aging. The algorithm makes use of the whole pattern in the brain image and additionally takes inter-regional dependencies into account (Bishop, 2006; Schölkopf and Smola, 2002). It further allows combining data from different MR scanners.

With an overall mean absolute (MAE) error of only 5 years and a correlation of $r = 0.92$ between chronological age and estimated brain age in a sample of 650 healthy subjects aged between 20 and 86 years (see chapter 2), this age estimating framework turned out to be a straightforward method to accurately and reliably estimate age with minimal preprocessing and parameter optimization. Additionally, in a recent study with a sample of about 400 healthy children and adolescents, aged 5 – 18 years, the *BrainAGE* framework performed even better, resulting in a MAE of only 1 year and a maturation curve that accounted for 87% sample variance (Franke et al., 2012b). Most remarkably, although brain maturation in childhood as well as brain aging in late life comprise very complex, multidimensional, and highly variable processes (Good et al., 2001; Lebel and Beaulieu, 2011; Lenroot and Giedd, 2006; Raz and Rodrigue, 2006; Resnick et al., 2003; Wilke and Holland, 2003), the confidence intervals of estimated brain age did not change as a function of age during brain maturation (Franke et al., 2012b) and brain aging (see chapter 2), underlining the potential of the approach to correctly capture the multidimensional characteristics of the different maturational and aging processes occurring in childhood and old age, respectively.

The amount of explained variance between chronological and estimated or predicted brain age as achieved by the presented *BrainAGE* approach was at least comparable or even better than by other approaches which provided a reverence curve for age-related brain changes using structural (Ashburner, 2007; Brown et al., 2012; Lao et al., 2004; Neeb et al., 2006) or functional (Dosenbach et al., 2010) MRI data. This holds true even though much less preprocessing and parameter optimization was used as compared to recent approaches (Brown et al., 2012; Dosenbach et al., 2010). Although it is conceivable that the combination of diverse data modalities (e.g., structural, functional, DTI) might achieve even higher prediction accuracies, the required multidimensional dataset would constitute a clear drawback. Additionally, structural imaging – in contrast to functional MRI – avoids potential biases due to diverse confounding influences (e.g., alertness, vigilance; Van Dijk et al., 2012) and already is the imaging modality of choice in most centers. Also, when using the *BrainAGE* method, multidimensional data appear to be not necessarily needed. Even more interesting, neither of the aforementioned approaches demonstrated the potential to provide diagnostic information in clinical samples.

Several variables were found to have the potential to influence the accuracy of age prediction, such as the number of subjects in the training sample, various parameters in data acquisition (e.g., field strength, scanning sequence) and data preprocessing (e.g., registration, smoothing), as well as the chosen approach to reduce data dimensionality (e.g., PCA; see chapters 2 and 3). Consequently, these variables need to be carefully controlled for in future studies. Even though, with intraclass correlations (ICC) up to 0.93 between the *BrainAGE* scores calculated from two shortly delayed scans and even across different MRI scanners, the *BrainAGE* framework proved its ability to provide very stable and reliable estimates (see chapter 3). Although sample-specific offsets in *BrainAGE* estimation sometimes emerge due to diverse parameters (e.g., kind of MRI scanner, field-strength, scanning sequences), those offsets can be easily corrected for by a linear shift, as they were systematic across subjects within the same sample. Consequently, when comparing *BrainAGE* scores in different clinical samples, a sample of healthy subjects should be included in order to control for a potential offset. On the other hand, if only differences in *BrainAGE* between two subsamples of the same sample or correlations to other measures are examined, there is no urgent need for the inclusion of control subjects and sample-specific offset correction.

When establishing a clinically valuable reference curve for structural age-related brain changes, an additional challenge is to develop an algorithm that allows combining data from different MRI scanners. The *BrainAGE* framework demonstrated strong stability of the estimated brain age, even with entirely new data that differed from the training data – not only by scanner but also by scanning parameters. Importantly, applying the *BrainAGE* method to data from scanners that were not included in the training step, the results proved to be reliable and moreover clinically valuable (see chapters 2 and 3; see also Franke et al., 2012b). Thus, with respect to combining data from different scanners and controlling for potential offsets, the *BrainAGE* framework proved to perform accurately, robustly, and even scanner-independently. These encouraging results are in line with (Klöppel et al., 2008b), indicating that the effect of scanner parameters is sufficiently different from that of the aging process, and that the *BrainAGE* method generalizes well across different scanners.

6.1.1 Limitations of the *BrainAGE* approach

It should be noted, that the *BrainAGE* approach was implemented to model a reference curve for "normal" structural brain maturation (Franke et al., 2012b) or brain aging (see chapter 2). Therefore, and in this stage of model development, the application to clinical samples is only recommended if the underlying disease is likely to result from overall deceleration or acceleration of brain maturation or brain aging, such as observed in subjects with developmental delays (Harbord et al., 1990; McLaughlin et al., 2010; Ramenghi et al., 2011; Verbruggen et al., 2009), schizophrenia (Kirkpatrick et al., 2008; Thompson et al., 2004), or Alzheimer's Disease (Bartzokis, 2011; Cao et al., 2010; Driscoll et al., 2009; Dukart et al., 2011; Jones et al., 2011; Saetre et al., 2011; Spulber et al., 2010; Thompson et al., 2004). Future work will extend and refine the current approach to allow identifying significant regional deviations from the expected age-specific pattern in order to provide region-specific information as a basis for further clinical applications.

Since diverse parameters were found to have the potential to influence the accuracy of age prediction (see chapters 2 and 3), the impact of varying image quality and segmentation quality in training and test data on brain age estimation quality could limit the reliability of the proposed method and thus should be carefully controlled in future studies. Additionally, they will be further analyzed within even larger samples.

One limitation of the *BrainAGE* approach might be that white matter lesions, which occur primarily due to cerebro-vascular diseases, are not detected in the segmentation approach. Those lesions are segmented as gray matter and might therefore influence the relevance vector regression. However, because such lesions only occur in a limited number of healthy subjects, whose data are used to build the reference curve for healthy brain aging, it is very unlikely that they contribute to the relevance vectors because of their high local variance. In future, the segmentation should be extended by methods that allow to detect white matter lesions even without any additional FLAIR sequence (Schwarz et al., 2009).

Several factors like cognitive reserve, education level, or socioeconomic status may protect subjects with anatomical signs of accelerated brain atrophy from developing AD and showing declining test performance, or could at least delay this process (Fotenos et al., 2008; Querbes et al., 2009; Snowdon, 2003). Consequently, subjects with high *BrainAGE* scores may not show AD-specific clinical symptoms yet, even though accelerated brain atrophy is already detectable at MRI. Future research will further investigate the relationship between cognitive reserve and *BrainAGE*.

Additionally, subjects with a high *BrainAGE* score but no AD-specific clinical profile may suffer from other neurodegenerative diseases. Depending on the availability of data, this issue should be explored by applying the *BrainAGE* method to other neurodegenerative diseases, i.e. predicting the severity of symptoms or the possible rate of decline of relevant clinical measures.

6.2 Application of the *BrainAGE* approach to clinical samples

As stated before, AD is widely believed to be a form of, or at least associated with, accelerated aging (Cao et al., 2010; Driscoll et al., 2009; Jones et al.,

2011; Saetre et al., 2011; Spulber et al., 2010; Thompson et al., 2004), with subtle structural brain changes accumulating over many years and dementia being the final stage (Frisoni et al., 2010; Jack et al., 2010). These processes may be caused by precocious and / or more pronounced myelin breakdown that leads to precocious and / or accelerated tissue loss, finally manifesting in severe disease pathology (Bartzokis, 2004, 2011; Bartzokis et al., 2012; Lu et al., 2011, 2013). In line with that, atrophied regions detected in AD patients were found to largely overlap with regions affected by "normal" age-related atrophy (Dukart et al., 2011).

The *BrainAGE* approach repeatedly proved its potential to indicate abnormal age-related neuroanatomical changes based on structural MRI data. Subjects with AD as well as MCI subjects who cognitively declined and converted to AD (i.e. pMCI) exhibited significantly larger baseline *BrainAGE* scores compared to control subjects as well as those with MCI who remained cognitively stable (i.e. sMCI; see chapters 3 and 5). Furthermore, the *BrainAGE* framework even proved its capability to recognize accelerated brain atrophy in a longitudinal design. Already starting with a significantly higher baseline *BrainAGE* score in pMCI and AD, age-related brain atrophy were shown to accelerate even more during follow-up. Compared to that, sMCI and healthy control subjects did not show any deviations from healthy brain aging at baseline or at follow-up. These results are in line with recent studies that showed increased GM atrophy in AD (Anderson et al., 2012), accelerated changes in whole brain volume in MCI (Driscoll et al., 2009), acceleration in atrophy rates as subjects progress from MCI to AD (Jack et al., 2008), and greater GM loss in certain regions in pMCI subjects (Ch'etelat et al., 2005; Desikan et al., 2008; Leow et al., 2009; McDonald et al., 2012; Sluimer et al., 2009). Additionally, the results further support the assumption of AD being a form of or at least being associated with accelerated age-related brain changes (Bartzokis, 2011; Cao et al., 2010; Driscoll et al., 2009; Dukart et al.,

2011; Jones et al., 2011; Saetre et al., 2011; Spulber et al., 2010; Thompson et al., 2004).

Even more interesting, acceleration in brain aging was found to be increased by about 4.5 years already in T2DM subjects as compared to non-diabetic controls (see chapter 4). Furthermore, the *BrainAGE* scores additionally increased in T2DM patients, but not in controls, during follow-up. This is in line with recent results, suggesting that T2DM leads to structural brain changes that show the pattern of accelerated aging (Araki et al., 1994; Biessels et al., 2006; Gispen and Biessels, 2000; Tan et al., 2011; van Elderen et al., 2010; Velayudhan et al., 2010), as well as further extends the body of evidence suggesting that acceleration in brain aging in T2DM is already quantifiable in a preclinical stage. Hence, the observed acceleration of brain atrophy in T2DM is likely to be associated with a precocious Alzheimerization (Bartzokis, 2011) and thus may reduce the threshold for developing dementia (Biessels et al., 2006).

Moreover, within this whole sample, those subjects with higher *BrainAGE* scores were more likely to consume more alcohol, which is in line with recent studies that claimed a U-shaped relationship between alcohol consumption and cognitive impairment (Anttila et al., 2004; Solfrizzi et al., 2008). Fasting blood glucose levels as a potential indicator of hyperglycemia, were also positively related to *BrainAGE* scores even in non-diabetic adults, supporting the notion about glucose-mediated accelerated brain aging in T2DM and even in the prediabetic state (Biessels et al., 2006; Tan et al., 2011). Even more interesting, increased $TNF\alpha$ levels, which were recently found to have a central role in the pathogenesis of AD (Tobinick and Gross, 2008), were also strongly related to higher *BrainAGE* scores. Consequently, future research will further explore the influences of health and lifestyle markers (e.g., metabolic syndrome, hypertension, nicotine and alcohol abuse, tHcy levels, vitamin B12 levels) on brain aging in cognitively non-impaired samples.

6.2.1 Associations of *BrainAGE* with cognitive functions

Although not specifically trained to predict changes in cognitive scales, individual *BrainAGE* scores were profoundly associated with measures of cognitive functioning as well as clinical disease severity in pMCI subjects and AD patients and even to its prospective worsening (see chapters 3 and 5). These results support the recently suggested relationship between progressive acceleration in brain aging and rate of cognitive decline as well as clinical disease severity in pMCI and AD samples (Desikan et al., 2008; Wilson et al., 2011).

Even more interesting, in pMCI subjects, accelerated brain aging was shown to be more closely related to the worsening of higher cognitive functions, whereas in AD patients, accelerated brain aging was more closely related to disease severity. However, the *BrainAGE* scores in healthy controls and sMCI subjects did not show significant correlations to measures cognitive functioning and disease severity. This may be mainly due to the fact that the scales analyzed in these studies were used specifically to identify clinical decline and deterioration in basic cognitive functioning in clinical samples. Consequently, future work will further explore the relationship between *BrainAGE* and higher cognitive functions, applying cognitive scales that are more appropriate to capture healthy cognitive aging.

Even in T2DM subjects without cognitive impairment, those with higher *BrainAGE* scores showed worse verbal fluency (see chapter 4). These results are consistent with previous findings that suggest subclinical cognitive impairment in T2DM and even in the prediabetic state (Baker et al., 2011; Tan et al., 2011; van Elderen et al., 2010). Finally, subjects with higher *BrainAGE* scores were also more likely to be depressed, which is line with recent studies that linked depression to a state of accelerated aging (Heuser, 2002; Wolkowitz et al., 2010, 2011) as well as showed an increased risk of dementia in patients with depression in general, and even worse in T2DM patients (Katon et al., 2012).

6.2.2 Prediction of prospective conversion to AD using *BrainAGE*

Predicting prospective worsening of cognitive functions and ultimately conversion to AD using the novel *BrainAGE* approach builds on the assumption that AD is preceded by an acceleration in brain atrophy, which resembles the structural brain changes seen in healthy brain aging, and thus is already quantifiable in a preclinical stage (e.g., Bartzokis, 2011; Cao et al., 2010; Driscoll et al., 2009; Dukart et al., 2011; Jones et al., 2011; Saetre et al., 2011; Spulber et al., 2010; Thompson et al., 2004). Consequently, the detection and quantification of abnormal (brain) changes is important for the prospective identification and subsequent treatment of individuals at risk for cognitive decline and dementia.

Although the best validated biomarkers for an early detection of AD include markers of brain Aβ-amyloid-plaque deposition (e.g., decreased CSF Aβ_{42}) as well as markers of neurodegeneration (e.g., increased CSF tau, decreased fluorodeoxyglucose uptake on PET (FDG-PET), and structural MRI measures of cerebral atrophy; Bartzokis, 2011; Jack et al., 2010), MRI was found to retain the closest relationship with cognitive decline (Jack et al., 2010; Vemuri et al., 2009a,b), suggesting a crucial role for structural MRI in predicting future conversion to AD (Frisoni et al., 2010; Jack et al., 2010). A recent longitudinal study provides additional support by reporting that those changes in brain structure occur several years before decline in cognitive functioning is measurable (Clark et al., 2012). Thus, the acceleration of spatiotemporal brain atrophy might only be seen in subjects in a preclinical stage, while in AD patients additional disease-specific pathological changes are occurring. In future research those age- and unrelated disease-based processes of brain tissue loss in AD should be disentangled.

Using high-dimensional pattern recognition with imaging data was recently suggested to provide a viable biomarker to detect subtle, but predictive, imaging phenotypes that precede cognitive decline while there is still opportunity for preventive or therapeutic interventions (Clark et al., 2012). Current classification approaches attempt to identify disease-specific patterns that allow a separation of subjects with MCI or AD from healthy samples. Whilst most approaches are able to accurately differentiate between healthy controls and AD patients (Hinrichs et al., 2011; Walhovd et al., 2010; Zhang et al., 2011), it is the conversion from MCI to AD that is of greater clinical interest and consequence, since individuals showing the first subtle signs of abnormal atrophy will benefit most from an early therapy.

In contrast to all existing approaches, the *BrainAGE* model aggregates the complex, multi-dimensional aging patterns across the whole brain and finally identifies abnormal brain atrophy in pMCI subjects prior to final conversion to AD, with increasing *BrainAGE* scores indicating an increased risk of developing AD. With accuracy rates up to 84% in predicting conversion to AD on an individual level up to three years in advance based on baseline MRI only (see chapter 5), the *BrainAGE* approach is in line with or even outperforms recent classification studies that predicted decline of cognitive scores in MCI subjects or short-term conversion to AD (Davatzikos et al., 2011; Fan et al., 2008a; Misra et al., 2009; Querbes et al., 2009; Teipel et al., 2007; Westman et al., 2011). Even more interestingly, a high *BrainAGE* score increased the prognostic certainty of a subsequent conversion to AD from 68% in the clinically defined MCI sample to 90%. This gain in certainty may provide solid diagnostic grounds for early intervention strategies aimed at delaying or preventing the onset of full-scale AD in subjects at highest risk for the disease.

Furthermore, the *BrainAGE* framework proved to be more precise in predicting conversion of MCI to AD when compared to chronological age, cognitive scores, hippocampus volume, or state-of-the-art CSF biomarkers. Although recent studies reported that combining MRI and CSF measures in a multivariate model resulted in better accuracy for predicting future conversion from MCI to AD than using either MRI or CSF separately (Westman et al., 2011), the *BrainAGE* approach, using only whole-brain structural baseline MRI, substantially improved classification accuracy and predictive power in detecting early AD. In contrast to CSF biomarkers, MRI is non-invasive and can be performed more rapidly than a detailed neuropsychological testing. Additionally, current models of the dynamics of well established biomarkers of the Alzheimer's pathological cascade suggest a crucial role for structural MRI in predicting future cognitive decline and conversion to AD, as MRI was shown to retain the closest relationship with memory loss as well as worsening of clinical functions (Clark et al., 2012; Frisoni et al., 2010; Jack et al., 2010). Even though hippocampus volume has been shown to represent an independent risk factor for AD and robustly predict conversion to AD in MCI subjects, the *BrainAGE* approach substantially outperformed prediction utilizing baseline hippocampus volumes within this study as well as recently published classification studies (Costafreda et al., 2011; Risacher et al., 2009, 2010).

Chapter 7.
Conclusions and perspectives

To summarize, the *BrainAGE* approach demonstrated its potential to provide a reliable, clinically sensitive, as well as easy-to-use reference curve of healthy brain aging. It was also repeatedly shown that this method can be applied to data from different scanners, which is an important prerequisite for use in clinical routines. Furthermore, the *BrainAGE* method has shown promising results on an individual level, contributing to an early indication of AD in advance of clinical symptoms, and even predicting prospective decline of clinical measures, thus probably facilitating early treatment or preventative interventions. Depending on data availability, future research could include application of the *BrainAGE* framework in order to evaluate therapeutic effects of drugs or other treatment modalities. Since diverse health and lifestyle factors were found to contribute to the risk of cognitive decline and even developing dementia, future explorations will apply the *BrainAGE* approach to subjects with the metabolic syndrome (Solfrizzi et al., 2011), or other lifestyle factors (Chen et al., 2009; Clarke, 2006; Scarmeas et al., 2009; Solfrizzi et al., 2008), to predict the severity of clinical symptoms or the rate of cognitive decline. Furthermore, the relationship between the duration of exposure to risk factors and accelerated brain aging, and whether reversal of modifiable factors might decelerate the progression of brain aging, should be investigated.

Additionally, the *BrainAGE* framework avoids time-consuming processing steps like manual segmentation and has already proven its ability to be efficiently used and to yield stable performance with multicenter studies as well as new test samples, unseen within the model training procedure. Furthermore, to train the *BrainAGE* algorithm for modeling the normal aging pattern, only a database of healthy, non-demented subjects is necessary. This is a unique, distinguishing feature compared to existing approaches that also need data of MCI and / or AD patients to predict cognitive decline or future conversion to AD.

Given that the *BrainAGE* framework is validated as well as fast and easy to use, this method holds great potential for application in daily clinical routine, especially since brain imaging has become part of the standard diagnostic work-up for many neuropsychiatric and neurodegenerative disorders.

References

Aizenstein, H. J., Nebes, R. D., Saxton, J. A., Price, J. C., Mathis, C. A., Tsopelas, N. D., Ziolko, S. K., James, J. A., Snitz, B. E., Houck, P. R., Bi, W., Cohen, A. D., Lopresti, B. J., DeKosky, S. T., Halligan, E. M., and Klunk, W. E. (2008). Frequent amyloid deposition without significant cognitive impairment among the elderly. *Archives of Neurology*, 65(11):1509–1517.

Albert, S. M. and Teresi, J. A. (1999). Reading ability, education, and cognitive status assessment among older adults in Harlem, New York City. *American Journal of Public Health*, 89(1):95– 97.

Alexander, G. E., Bergfield, K. L., Chen, K., Reiman, E. M., Hanson, K. D., Lin, L., Bandy, D., Caselli, R. J., and Moeller, J. R. (2012). Gray matter network associated with risk for Alzheimer's disease in young to middle-aged adults. *Neurobiology of Aging*, 33(12):2723–2732.

Alexander, G. E., Furey, M. L., Grady, C. L., Pietrini, P., Brady, D. R., Mentis, M. J., and Schapiro, M. B. (1997). Association of premorbid intellectual function with cerebral metabolism in Alzheimer's disease: implications for the cognitive reserve hypothesis. *American Journal of Psychiatry*, 154(2):165–172.

Ali, S., Stone, M. A., Peters, J. L., Davies, M. J., and Khunti, K. (2006). The prevalence of comorbid depression in adults with type 2 diabetes: a systematic review and meta-analysis. *Diabetic Medicine*, 23(11):1165–1173.

Anderson, R. J., Freedland, K. E., Clouse, R. E., and Lustman, P. J. (2001). The prevalence of comorbid depression in adults with diabetes: a meta-analysis. *Diabetes Care*, 24(6):1069–1078.

Anderson, V. M., Schott, J. M., Bartlett, J. W., Leung, K. K., Miller, D. H., and Fox, N. C. (2012). Gray matter atrophy rate as a marker of disease progression in AD. *Neurobiology of Aging*, 33(7):1194–1202.

Anttila, T., Helkala, E.-L., Viitanen, M., Kareholt, I., Fratiglioni, L., Winblad, B., Soininen, H., Tuomilehto, J., Nissinen, A., and Kivipelto, M. (2004). Alcohol drinking in middle age and subsequent risk of mild cognitive impairment and dementia in old age: a prospective population based study. *BMJ*, 329(7465):539.

Araki, Y., Nomura, M., Tanaka, H., Yamamoto, H., Yamamoto, T., Tsukaguchi, I., and Nakamura, H. (1994). MRI of the brain in diabetes mellitus. *Neuroradiology*, 36(2):101–103.

Artero, S., Tiemeier, H., Prins, N. D., Sabatier, R., Breteler, M. M. B., and Ritchie, K. (2004). Neuroanatomical localisation and clinical correlates of white matter lesions in the elderly. *Journal of Neurology, Neurosurgery, and Psychiatry*, 75(9):1304–1308.

Ashburner, J. (2007). A fast diffeomorphic image registration algorithm. *Neuroimage*, 38(1):95–113.

Ashburner, J. (2009). Computational anatomy with the SPM software. *Magnetic Resonance Imaging*, 27(8):1163–1174.

Ashburner, J., Csernansky, J. G., Davatzikos, C., Fox, N. C., Frisoni, G. B., and Thompson, P. M. (2003). Computer-assisted imaging to assess brain structure in healthy and diseased brains. *Lancet Neurology*, 2(2):79–88.

Ashburner, J. and Friston, K. J. (2000). Voxel-based morphometry – the methods. *Neuroimage*, 11(6):805–821.

Ashburner, J. and Friston, K. J. (2005). Unified segmentation. *Neuroimage*, 26(3):839–51.

Baker, L. D., Cross, D. J., Minoshima, S., Belongia, D., Watson, G. S., and Craft, S. (2011). Insulin resistance and Alzheimer-like reductions in regional cerebral glucose metabolism for cognitively normal adults with prediabetes or early type 2 diabetes. *Archives of Neurology*, 68(1):51–57.

Bartzokis, G. (2004). Age-related myelin breakdown: a developmental model of cognitive decline and Alzheimer's disease. *Neurobiology of Aging*, 25(1):5–18.

Bartzokis, G. (2011). Alzheimer's disease as homeostatic responses to age-related myelin breakdown. *Neurobiology of Aging*, 32(8):1341–1371.

Bartzokis, G., Lu, P. H., Heydari, P., Couvrette, A., Lee, G. J., Kalashyan, G., Freeman, F., Grinstead, J. W., Villablanca, P., Finn, J. P., Mintz, J., Alger, J. R., and Altshuler, L. L. (2012). Multimodal magnetic resonance imaging assessment of white matter aging trajectories over the lifespan of healthy individuals. *Biological Psychiatry*, 72(12):1026–1034.

Bennett, K. P. and Campbell, C. (2003). Support vector machines: hype or hallelujah? *SIGKDD Explorations*, 2:1–13.

Bertoni-Freddari, C., Fattoretti, P., Delfino, A., Solazzi, M., Giorgetti, B., Ulrich, J., and Meier-Ruge, W. (2002). Deafferentative synaptopathology in physiological aging and Alzheimer's disease. *Annals of the New York Academy of Sciences*, 977:322–326.

Biessels, G. J., Staekenborg, S., Brunner, E., Brayne, C., and Scheltens, P. (2006). Risk of dementia in diabetes mellitus: a systematic review. *Lancet Neurology*, 5(1):64–74.

Bishop, C. (2006). *Pattern Recognition and Machine Learning*. Springer, New York, NY.

Bookheimer, S. Y., Strojwas, M. H., Cohen, M. S., Saunders, A. M., Pericak-Vance, M. A., Mazziotta, J. C., and Small, G. W. (2000). Patterns of brain activation in people at risk for Alzheimer's disease. *New England Journal of Medicine*, 343(7):450–456.

Braak, H. and Braak, E. (1996). Development of Alzheimer-related neurofibrillary changes in the neocortex inversely recapitulates cortical myelogenesis. *Acta Neuropathologica*, 92(2):197–201.

Brant-Zawadzki, M., Weinstein, P., Bartkowski, H., and Moseley, M. (1987). MR imaging and spectroscopy in clinical and experimental cerebral ischemia: a review. *American Journal of Roentgenology*, 148(3):579–588.

Brookmeyer, R., Johnson, E., Ziegler-Graham, K., and Arrighi, H. M. (2007). Forecasting the global burden of Alzheimer's disease. *Alzheimer's & Dementia*, 3(3):186–191.

Brown, T. T., Kuperman, J. M., Chung, Y., Erhart, M., McCabe, C., Hagler, Jr, D. J., Venka- traman, V. K., Akshoomoff, N., Amaral, D. G., Bloss, C. S., Casey, B. J., Chang, L., Ernst, T. M.,

Frazier, J. A., Gruen, J. R., Kaufmann, W. E., Kenet, T., Kennedy, D. N., Murray, S. S., Sowell, E. R., Jernigan, T. L., and Dale, A. M. (2012). Neuroanatomical assessment of biological maturity. *Current Biology*, 22(18):1693–1698.

Brown, W. R., Moody, D. M., Challa, V. R., Thore, C. R., and Anstrom, J. A. (2002). Venous collagenosis and arteriolar tortuosity in leukoaraiosis. *Journal of the Neurological Sciences*, 203-204:159–163.

Buchhave, P., Minthon, L., Zetterberg, H., Wallin, A. K., Blennow, K., and Hansson, O. (2012). Cerebrospinal fluid levels of β-amyloid 1-42, but not of tau, are fully changed already 5 to 10 years before the onset of Alzheimer dementia. *Archives of General Psychiatry*, 69(1):98–106.

Cao, K., Chen-Plotkin, A. S., Plotkin, J. B., and Wang, L.-S. (2010). Age-correlated gene expression in normal and neurodegenerative human brain tissues. *PLoS One*, 5(9):e13098.

Carmelli, D., Swan, G. E., Reed, T., Wolf, P. A., Miller, B. L., and DeCarli, C. (1999). Midlife cardiovascular risk factors and brain morphology in identical older male twins. *Neurology*, 52(6):1119–1124.

Chalimourda, A., Schölkopf, B., and Smola, A. J. (2004). Experimentally optimal nu in support vector regression for different noise models and parameter settings. *Neural Networks*, 17(1):127–141.

Chen, J.-H., Lin, K.-P., and Chen, Y.-C. (2009). Risk factors for dementia. *Journal of the Formosan Medical Association*, 108(10):754–764.

Cheng, G., Huang, C., Deng, H., and Wang, H. (2012). Diabetes as a risk factor for dementia and mild cognitive impairment: a meta-analysis of longitudinal studies. *Internal Medicine Journal*, 42(5):484–491.

Cherkassky, V. and Ma, Y. (2004). Practical selection of SVM parameters and noise estimation for SVM regression. *Neural Networks*, 17(1):113–126.

Chételat, G., Landeau, B., Eustache, F., Mézenge, F., Viader, F., de la Sayette, V., Desgranges, B., and Baron, J.-C. (2005). Using voxel-based morphometry to map the structural changes associated with rapid conversion in MCI: a longitudinal MRI study. *Neuroimage*, 27(4):934–946.

Clark, C. M., Xie, S., Chittams, J., Ewbank, D., Peskind, E., Galasko, D., Morris, J. C., McKeel, Jr, D. W., Farlow, M., Weitlauf, S. L., Quinn, J., Kaye, J., Knopman, D., Arai, H., Doody, R. S., DeCarli, C., Leight, S., Lee, V. M.-Y., and Trojanowski, J. Q. (2003). Cerebrospinal fluid tau and beta-amyloid: how well do these biomarkers reflect autopsy-confirmed dementia diagnoses? *Archives of Neurology*, 60(12):1696–1702.

Clark, V. H., Resnick, S. M., Doshi, J., Beason-Held, L. L., Zhou, Y., Ferrucci, L., Wong, D. F., Kraut, M. A., and Davatzikos, C. (2012). Longitudinal imaging pattern analysis (SPARE-CD index) detects early structural and functional changes before cognitive decline in healthy older adults. *Neurobiology of Aging*, 33(12):2733–2745.

Clarke, R. (2006). Vitamin B12, folic acid, and the prevention of dementia. *New England Journal of Medicine*, 354(26):2817–2819.

Clarke, R., Birks, J., Nexo, E., Ueland, P. M., Schneede, J., Scott, J., Molloy, A., and Evans, J. G. (2007). Low vitamin B-12 status and risk of cognitive decline in older adults. *American Journal of Clinical Nutrition*, 86(5):1384–1391.

Clarke, R., Smith, A. D., Jobst, K. A., Refsum, H., Sutton, L., and Ueland, P. M. (1998). Folate, vitamin B12, and serum total homocysteine levels in confirmed Alzheimer disease. *Archives of Neurology*, 55(11):1449–1455.

Cockrell, J. R. and Folstein, M. F. (1988). Mini-mental state examination (MMSE). Psychopharmacology Bulletin, 24(4):689–692.

Cook, I. A., Leuchter, A. F., Morgan, M. L., Dunkin, J. J., Witte, E., David, S., Mickes, L., O'Hara, R., Simon, S., Lufkin, R., Abrams, M., and Rosenberg, S. (2004). Longitudinal progression of subclinical structural brain disease in normal aging. *American Journal of Geriatric Psychiatry*, 12(2):190–200.

Cosentino, S., Scarmeas, N., Helzner, E., Glymour, M. M., Brandt, J., Albert, M., Blacker, D., and Stern, Y. (2008). APOE epsilon 4 allele predicts faster cognitive decline in mild Alzheimer disease. *Neurology*, 70(19):1842–1849.

Costafreda, S. G., Dinov, I. D., Tu, Z., Shi, Y., Liu, C.-Y., Kloszewska, I., Mecocci, P., Soininen, H., Tsolaki, M., Vellas, B., Wahlund, L.-O., Spenger, C., Toga, A. W., Lovestone, S., and Simmons, A. (2011). Automated hippocampal shape analysis predicts the onset of dementia in mild cognitive impairment. *Neuroimage*, 56(1):212–219.

Cuadra, M. B., Cammoun, L., Butz, T., Cuisenaire, O., and Thiran, J.-P. (2005). Comparison and validation of tissue modelization and statistical classification methods in T1-weighted MR brain images. *IEEE Transactions on Medical Imaging*, 24(12):1548–1565.

Davatzikos, C., Bhatt, P., Shaw, L. M., Batmanghelich, K. N., and Trojanowski, J. Q. (2011). Prediction of MCI to AD conversion, via MRI, CSF biomarkers, and pattern classification. *Neurobiology of Aging*, 32(12):2322.e19–27.

Davatzikos, C., Fan, Y., Wu, X., Shen, D., and Resnick, S. M. (2008a). Detection of prodromal Alzheimer's disease via pattern classification of magnetic resonance imaging. *Neurobiology of Aging*, 29(4):514–523.

Davatzikos, C., Resnick, S. M., Wu, X., Parmpi, P., and Clark, C. M. (2008b). Individual patient diagnosis of AD and FTD via high-dimensional pattern classification of MRI. *Neuroimage*, 41(4):1220–1227.

Davatzikos, C., Shen, D., Gur, R. C., Wu, X., Liu, D., Fan, Y., Hughett, P., Turetsky, B. I., and Gur, R. E. (2005). Whole-brain morphometric study of schizophrenia revealing a spatially complex set of focal abnormalities. *Archives of General Psychiatry*, 62(11):1218–1227.

Davatzikos, C., Xu, F., An, Y., Fan, Y., and Resnick, S. M. (2009). Longitudinal progression of Alzheimer's-like patterns of atrophy in normal older adults: the SPARE-AD index. *Brain*, 132(8):2026–2035.

de Bresser, J., Tiehuis, A. M., van den Berg, E., Reijmer, Y. D., Jongen, C., Kappelle, L. J., Mali, W. P., Viergever, M. A., Biessels, G. J., and Utrecht Diabetic Encephalopathy Study Group (2010). Progression of cerebral atrophy and white matter hyperintensities in patients with type 2 diabetes. *Diabetes Care*, 33(6):1309–1314.

De Leeuw, F. E., De Groot, J. C., and Breteler, M. M. B. (2001). White matter changes: frequency and risk factors. In Pantoni, L., Inzitari, D., and Wallin, A., editors, *The Matter of White Matter: Clinical and Pathophysiological Aspects of White Matter Disease Related to Cognitive Decline and Vascular Dementia*, pages 19 – 33. Academic Pharmaceutical Productions, Utrecht, The Netherlands.

de Leon, M. J., Convit, A., Wolf, O. T., Tarshish, C. Y., DeSanti, S., Rusinek, H., Tsui, W., Kandil, E., Scherer, A. J., Roche, A., Imossi, A., Thorn, E., Bobinski, M., Caraos, C., Lesbre, P., Schlyer, D., Poirier, J., Reisberg, B., and Fowler, J. (2001). Prediction of cognitive decline in normal elderly subjects with 2-[(18)F]fluoro-2-deoxy-D-glucose / positron-emission tomography (FDG/PET). *Proceedings of the National Academy of Sciences of the United States of America*, 98(19):10966–10971.

Deary, I. J., Whiteman, M. C., Pattie, A., Starr, J. M., Hayward, C., Wright, A. F., Carothers, A., and Whalley, L. J. (2002). Cognitive change and the APOE epsilon 4 allele. *Nature*, 418(6901):932.

Debette, S., Beiser, A., Hoffmann, U., Decarli, C., O'Donnell, C. J., Massaro, J. M., Au, R., Himali, J. J., Wolf, P. A., Fox, C. S., and Seshadri, S. (2010). Visceral fat is associated with lower brain volume in healthy middle-aged adults. *Annals of Neurology*, 68(2):136–144.

den Heijer, T., Launer, L. J., Prins, N. D., van Dijk, E. J., Vermeer, S. E., Hofman, A., Koudstaal, P. J., and Breteler, M. M. B. (2005). Association between blood pressure, white matter lesions, and atrophy of the medial temporal lobe. *Neurology*, 64(2):263–267.

Desikan, R. S., Fischl, B., Cabral, H. J., Kemper, T. L., Guttmann, C. R. G., Blacker, D., Hyman, B. T., Albert, M. S., and Killiany, R. J. (2008). MRI measures of temporoparietal regions show differential rates of atrophy during prodromal AD. *Neurology*, 71(11):819–825.

Donix, M., Ercoli, L. M., Siddarth, P., Brown, J. A., Martin-Harris, L., Burggren, A. C., Miller, K. J., Small, G. W., and Bookheimer, S. Y. (2012). Influence of Alzheimer disease family history and genetic risk on cognitive performance in healthy middle-aged and older people. *The American Journal of Geriatric Psychiatry*, 20(7):565–573.

Dosenbach, N. U. F., Nardos, B., Cohen, A. L., Fair, D. A., Power, J. D., Church, J. A., Nelson, S. M., Wig, G. S., Vogel, A. C., Lessov-Schlaggar, C. N., Barnes, K. A., Dubis, J. W., Feczko, E., Coalson, R. S., Pruett, Jr, J. R., Barch, D. M., Petersen, S. E., and Schlaggar, B. L. (2010). Prediction of individual brain maturity using fMRI. *Science*, 329(5997):1358–1361.

Driscoll, I., Davatzikos, C., An, Y., Wu, X., Shen, D., Kraut, M., and Resnick, S. M. (2009). Longitudinal pattern of regional brain volume change differentiates normal aging from MCI. *Neurology*, 72(22):1906–1913.

Du, A.-T., Schuff, N., Chao, L. L., Kornak, J., Jagust, W. J., Kramer, J. H., Reed, B. R., Miller, B. L., Norman, D., Chui, H. C., and Weiner, M. W. (2006). Age effects on atrophy rates of entorhinal cortex and hippocampus. *Neurobiology of Aging*, 27(5):733–740.

Du, A. T., Schuff, N., Zhu, X. P., Jagust, W. J., Miller, B. L., Reed, B. R., Kramer, J. H., Mungas, D., Yaffe, K., Chui, H. C., and Weiner, M. W. (2003). Atrophy rates of entorhinal cortex in AD and normal aging. *Neurology*, 60(3):481–486.

Duchesnay, E., Cachia, A., Roche, A., Rivière, D., Cointepas, Y., Papadopoulos-Orfanos, D., Zilbovicius, M., Martinot, J.-L., Régis, J., and Mangin, J.-F. (2007). Classification based on cortical folding patterns. *IEEE Transactions on Medical Imaging*, 26(4):553–565.

Duchesne, S., Caroli, A., Geroldi, C., Collins, D. L., and Frisoni, G. B. (2009). Relating one-year cognitive change in mild cognitive impairment to baseline MRI features. *Neuroimage*, 47(4):1363–1370.

Dukart, J., Schroeter, M. L., Mueller, K., and Alzheimer's Disease Neuroimaging Initiative (2011). Age correction in dementia-matching to a healthy brain. *PLoS One*, 6(7):e22193.

Ellinson, M., Thomas, J., and Patterson, A. (2004). A critical evaluation of the relationship between serum vitamin B, folate and total homocysteine with cognitive impairment in the elderly. *Journal of Human Nutrition and Dietetics*, 17(4):371–383.

Ellis, R. S. (1920). Norms for some structural changes in the human cerebellum from birth to old age. *Journal of Comparative Neurology*, 32(1):1–33.

Enzinger, C., Fazekas, F., Matthews, P. M., Ropele, S., Schmidt, H., Smith, S., and Schmidt, R. (2005). Risk factors for progression of brain atrophy in aging: six-year follow-up of normal subjects. *Neurology*, 64(10):1704–1711.

Erickson, K. I., Raji, C. A., Lopez, O. L., Becker, J. T., Rosano, C., Newman, A. B., Gach, H. M., Thompson, P. M., Ho, A. J., and Kuller, L. H. (2010). Physical activity predicts gray matter volume in late adulthood: the Cardiovascular Health Study. *Neurology*, 75(16):1415–1422.

Evans, D. A., Beckett, L. A., Albert, M. S., Hebert, L. E., Scherr, P. A., Funkenstein, H. H., and Taylor, J. O. (1993). Level of education and change in cognitive function in a community population of older persons. *Annals of Epidemiology*, 3(1):71–77.

Ewers, M., Frisoni, G. B., Teipel, S. J., Grinberg, L. T., Amaro, Jr, E., Heinsen, H., Thompson, P. M., and Hampel, H. (2011). Staging Alzheimer's disease progression with multimodality neuroimaging. *Progress in Neurobiology*, 95(4):535–546.

Fan, Y., Batmanghelich, N., Clark, C. M., Davatzikos, C., and Alzheimer's Disease Neuroimaging Initiative (2008a). Spatial patterns of brain atrophy in MCI patients, identified via high-dimensional pattern classification, predict subsequent cognitive decline. *Neuroimage*, 39(4):1731–1743.

Fan, Y., Resnick, S. M., Wu, X., and Davatzikos, C. (2008b). Structural and functional biomarkers of prodromal Alzheimer's disease: a high-dimensional pattern classification study. *Neuroimage*, 41(2):277–285.

Faul, A. and Tipping, M. (2002). Analysis of sparse bayesian learning. In Dietterich, T. G., Becker, S., and Ghahramani, Z., editors, *Advances in Neural Information Processing Systems 14*, pages 383–389. MIT Press.

Fazekas, F., Ropele, S., Enzinger, C., Gorani, F., Seewann, A., Petrovic, K., and Schmidt, R. (2005). MTI of white matter hyperintensities. *Brain*, 128(12):2926–2932.

Féart, C., Samieri, C., and Barberger-Gateau, P. (2010). Mediterranean diet and cognitive function in older adults. *Current Opinion in Clinical Nutrition and Metabolic Care*, 13(1):14–18.

Filippini, N., Rao, A., Wetten, S., Gibson, R. A., Borrie, M., Guzman, D., Kertesz, A., Loy- English, I., Williams, J., Nichols, T., Whitcher, B., and Matthews, P. M. (2009). Anatomically-distinct genetic associations of APOE epsilon4 allele load with regional cortical atrophy in Alzheimer's disease. *Neuroimage*, 44(3):724–728.

Fisher, N. J., Tierney, M. C., Rourke, B. P., and Szalai, J. P. (2004). Verbal fluency patterns in two subgroups of patients with Alzheimer's disease. *The Clinical Neuropsychologist*, 18(1):122–131.

Fitzpatrick, A. L., Kuller, L. H., Lopez, O. L., Diehr, P., O'Meara, E. S., Longstreth, Jr, W. T., and Luchsinger, J. A. (2009). Midlife and late-life obesity and the risk of dementia: cardio- vascular health study. *Archives of Neurology*, 66(3):336–342.

Fotenos, A. F., Mintun, M. A., Snyder, A. Z., Morris, J. C., and Buckner, R. L. (2008). Brain volume decline in aging: evidence for a relation between socioeconomic status, preclinical Alzheimer disease, and reserve. *Archives of Neurology*, 65(1):113–120.

Franke, K., Gaser, C., and Alzheimer's Disease Neuroimaging Initiative (2012a). Longitudinal changes in individual *BrainAGE* in healthy aging, mild cognitive impairment, and Alzheimer's disease. *GeroPsych*, 25(4):235–245.

Franke, K., Gaser, C., Manor, B., and Novak, V. (2013a). Advanced *BrainAGE* in older adults with type 2 diabetes mellitus. *Frontiers in Aging Neuroscience*, 5(90):doi: 10.3389/fnagi.2013.00090.

Franke, K., Luders, E., May, A., Wilke, M., and Gaser, C. (2012b). Brain maturation: predicting individual *BrainAGE* in children and adolescents using structural MRI. *Neuroimage*, 63(3):1305–1312.

Franke, K., Ristow, M., and Gaser, C. (2013b). Gender-specific effects of health and lifestyle markers on individual *BrainAGE*. In *2013 International Workshop on Pattern Recognition in Neuroimaging (PRNI), IEEE Conference Proceedings*, pages 94–97.

Franke, K., Ziegler, G., Klöppel, S., Gaser, C., and Alzheimer's Disease Neuroimaging Initiative (2010). Estimating the age of healthy subjects from T1-weighted MRI scans using kernel methods: exploring the influence of various parameters. *Neuroimage*, 50(3):883–892.

Frisardi, V., Panza, F., Seripa, D., Imbimbo, B. P., Vendemiale, G., Pilotto, A., and Solfrizzi, V. (2010). Nutraceutical properties of mediterranean diet and cognitive decline: possible underlying mechanisms. *Journal of Alzheimer's Disease*, 22(3):715–740.

Frisoni, G. B., Fox, N. C., Jack, Jr, C. R., Scheltens, P., and Thompson, P. M. (2010). The clinical use of structural MRI in Alzheimer disease. *Nature Reviews Neurology*, 6(2):67–77.

Garratt, A., Schmidt, L., Mackintosh, A., and Fitzpatrick, R. (2002). Quality of life measurement: bibliographic study of patient assessed health outcome measures. *BMJ*, 324(7351):1417.

Gaser, C. (2009). Partial volume segmentation with Adaptive Maximum a Posteriori (MAP) approach. *Neuroimage*, 47:S121.

Gaser, C., Franke, K., Klöppel, S., Koutsouleris, N., Sauer, H., and Alzheimer's Disease Neuroimaging Initiative (2013). *BrainAGE* in mild cognitive impaired patients: Predicting the conversion to Alzheimer's disease. *PLoS One*, 8(6):e67346.

Gaser, C., Volz, H. P., Kiebel, S., Riehemann, S., and Sauer, H. (1999). Detecting structural changes in whole brain based on nonlinear deformations-application to schizophrenia research. *Neuroimage*, 10(2):107–113.

Ghosh, Subimal Ghosh, S. and Mujumdar, P. P. (2008). Statistical downscaling of GCM simulations to streamflow using relevance vector machine. *Advances in Water Resources*, 31(1):132–146.

Giedd, J. N., Lalonde, F. M., Celano, M. J., White, S. L., Wallace, G. L., Lee, N. R., and Lenroot, R. K. (2009). Anatomical brain magnetic resonance imaging of typically developing children and adolescents. *Journal of the American Academy of Child and Adolescent Psychiatry*, 48(5):465–470.

Gispen, W. H. and Biessels, G. J. (2000). Cognition and synaptic plasticity in diabetes mellitus. *Trends in Neurosciences*, 23(11):542–549.

Gogtay, N., Giedd, J. N., Lusk, L., Hayashi, K. M., Greenstein, D., Vaituzis, A. C., Nugent, 3rd, T. F., Herman, D. H., Clasen, L. S., Toga, A. W., Rapoport, J. L., and Thompson, P. M. (2004). Dynamic mapping of human cortical development during childhood through early adulthood. *Proceedings of the National Academy of Sciences USA*, 101(21):8174–8179.

Gogtay, N. and Thompson, P. M. (2010). Mapping gray matter development: implications for typical development and vulnerability to psychopathology. *Brain and Cognition*, 72(1):6–15.

Goldstein, I. B., Bartzokis, G., Guthrie, D., and Shapiro, D. (2002). Ambulatory blood pressure and brain atrophy in the healthy elderly. *Neurology*, 59(5):713–719.

Good, C. D., Johnsrude, I. S., Ashburner, J., Henson, R. N., Friston, K. J., and Frackowiak, R. S. (2001). A voxel-based morphometric study of ageing in 465 normal adult human brains. *Neuroimage*, 14(1):21–36.

Gu, Y., Nieves, J. W., Stern, Y., Luchsinger, J. A., and Scarmeas, N. (2010). Food combination and Alzheimer disease risk: a protective diet. *Archives of Neurology*, 67(6):699–706.

Gunning-Dixon, F. M. and Raz, N. (2003). Neuroanatomical correlates of selected executive functions in middle-aged and older adults: a prospective MRI study. *Neuropsychologia*, 41(14):1929–1941.

Guyon, I. and Elisseeff, A. (2003). An introduction to variable and feature selection. *Journal of Machine Learning Research*, 3:1157–1182.

Guyon, I., Weston, J., Barnhill, S., and Vapnik, V. (2002). Gene selection for cancer classification using support vector machines. *Machine Learning*, 46:389–422.

Hadjidemetriou, S., Lorenzen, P., Schuff, N., Mueller, S., and Weiner, M. (2008). Computational atlases of severity of white matter lesions in elderly subjects with MRI. *Medical Image Computing and Computer-Assisted Intervention (MICCAI)*, 11(Pt 1):450–458.

Harbord, M. G., Finn, J. P., Hall-Craggs, M. A., Robb, S. A., Kendall, B. E., and Boyd, S. G. (1990). Myelination patterns on magnetic resonance of children with developmental delay. *Developmental Medicine and Child Neurology*, 32(4):295–303.

Harris, S. E. and Deary, I. J. (2011). The genetics of cognitive ability and cognitive ageing in healthy older people. *Trends in Cognitive Sciences*, 15(9):388–394.

Harrison, J. E., Buxton, P., Husain, M., and Wise, R. (2000). Short test of semantic and phonological fluency: normal performance, validity and test-retest reliability. *The British Journal of Clinical Psychology*, 39 (Pt 2):181–191.

Heise, V., Filippini, N., Ebmeier, K. P., and Mackay, C. E. (2011). The APOE ε4 allele modulates brain white matter integrity in healthy adults. *Molecular Psychiatry*, 16(9):908–916.

Hesse, C., Rosengren, L., Andreasen, N., Davidsson, P., Vanderstichele, H., Vanmechelen, E., and Blennow, K. (2001). Transient increase in total tau but not phospho-tau in human cerebrospinal fluid after acute stroke. *Neuroscience Letters*, 297(3):187–190.

Heuser, I. (2002). Depression, endocrinologically a syndrome of premature aging? *Maturitas*, 41 Suppl 1:S19–23.

Hinrichs, C., Singh, V., Xu, G., Johnson, S. C., and Alzheimers Disease Neuroimaging Initiative (2011). Predictive markers for AD in a multi-modality framework: an analysis of MCI progression in the ADNI population. *Neuroimage*, 55(2):574–589.

Holm, S. (1979). A simple sequentially rejective multiple test procedure. *Scandinavian Journal of Statistics*, 6:65–70.

Holmes, D. (1990). The robustness of the usual correction for restriction in range due to explicit selection. *Psychometrika*, 55:19–32.

Jack, Jr, C. R., Knopman, D. S., Jagust, W. J., Shaw, L. M., Aisen, P. S., Weiner, M. W., Petersen, R. C., and Trojanowski, J. Q. (2010). Hypothetical model of dynamic biomarkers of the Alzheimer's pathological cascade. *Lancet Neurology*, 9(1):119–128.

Jack, Jr, C. R., Lowe, V. J., Weigand, S. D., Wiste, H. J., Senjem, M. L., Knopman, D. S., Shiung, M. M., Gunter, J. L., Boeve, B. F., Kemp, B. J., Weiner, M., Petersen, R. C., and Alzheimer's Disease Neuroimaging Initiative (2009). Serial PIB and MRI in normal, mild cognitive impairment and Alzheimer's disease: implications for sequence of pathological events in Alzheimer's disease. *Brain*, 132(5):1355–1365.

Jack, Jr, C. R., Weigand, S. D., Shiung, M. M., Przybelski, S. A., O'Brien, P. C., Gunter, J. L., Knopman, D. S., Boeve, B. F., Smith, G. E., and Petersen, R. C. (2008). Atrophy rates accelerate in amnestic mild cognitive impairment. *Neurology*, 70(19):1740–1752.

Jacobs, B., Driscoll, L., and Schall, M. (1997). Life-span dendritic and spine changes in areas 10 and 18 of human cortex: a quantitative Golgi study. *Journal of Comparative Neurology*, 386(4):661–680.

Janson, J., Laedtke, T., Parisi, J. E., O'Brien, P., Petersen, R. C., and Butler, P. C. (2004). Increased risk of type 2 diabetes in Alzheimer disease. *Diabetes*, 53(2):474–481.

Jones, D. T., Machulda, M. M., Vemuri, P., McDade, E. M., Zeng, G., Senjem, M. L., Gunter, J. L., Przybelski, S. A., Avula, R. T., Knopman, D. S., Boeve, B. F., Petersen, R. C., and Jack, Jr, C. R. (2011). Age-related changes in the default mode network are more advanced in Alzheimer disease. *Neurology*, 77(16):1524–1531.

Josephs, K. A., Whitwell, J. L., Ahmed, Z., Shiung, M. M., Weigand, S. D., Knopman, D. S., Boeve, B. F., Parisi, J. E., Petersen, R. C., Dickson, D. W., and Jack, Jr, C. R. (2008). Beta-amyloid burden is not associated with rates of brain atrophy. *Annals of Neurology*, 63(2):204–212.

Kadota, T., Horinouchi, T., and Kuroda, C. (2001). Development and aging of the cerebrum: assessment with proton MR spectroscopy. *American Journal of Neuroradiology*, 22(1):128–135.

Katon, W., Lyles, C. R., Parker, M. M., Karter, A. J., Huang, E. S., and Whitmer, R. A. (2012). Association of depression with increased risk of dementia in patients with type 2 diabetes: the Diabetes and Aging Study. *Archives of General Psychiatry*, 69(4):410–417.

Katzman, R., Aronson, M., Fuld, P., Kawas, C., Brown, T., Morgenstern, H., Frishman, W., Gidez, L., Eder, H., and Ooi, W. L. (1989). Development of dementing illnesses in an 80-year-old volunteer cohort. *Annals of Neurology*, 25(4):317–324.

Kemper, T. L. (1994). Neuroanatomical and neuropathological changes during aging and dementia. In Albert, M. L. and Knoefel, J. E., editors, *Clinical neurology of aging*, pages 3–67. Oxford University Press, New York, 2nd edition.

Kennedy, K. M. and Raz, N. (2005). Age, sex and regional brain volumes predict perceptual-motor skill acquisition. *Cortex*, 41(4):560–569.

Kidwell, C. S., el Saden, S., Livshits, Z., Martin, N. A., Glenn, T. C., and Saver, J. L. (2001). Transcranial Doppler pulsatility indices as a measure of diffuse small-vessel disease. *Journal of Neuroimaging*, 11(3):229–235.

Kirkpatrick, B., Messias, E., Harvey, P. D., Fernandez-Egea, E., and Bowie, C. R. (2008). Is schizophrenia a syndrome of accelerated aging? *Schizophrenia Bulletin*, 34(6):1024–1032.

Klöppel, S., Abdulkadir, A., Hadjidemetriou, S., Issleib, S., Frings, L., Thanh, T. N., Mader, I., Teipel, S. J., Hu´ll, M., and Ronneberger, O. (2011). A comparison of different automated methods for the detection of white matter lesions in MRI data. *Neuroimage*, 57(2):416–422.

Klöppel, S., Chu, C., Tan, G. C., Draganski, B., Johnson, H., Paulsen, J. S., Kienzle, W., Tabrizi, S. J., Ashburner, J., Frackowiak, R. S. J., and PREDICT-HD Investigators of the Huntington Study Group (2009). Automatic detection of preclinical neurodegeneration: presymptomatic Huntington disease. *Neurology*, 72(5):426–431.

Klöppel, S., Stonnington, C. M., Barnes, J., Chen, F., Chu, C., Good, C. D., Mader, I., Mitchell, L. A., Patel, A. C., Roberts, C. C., Fox, N. C., Jack, Jr, C. R., Ashburner, J., and Frackowiak, R. S. J. (2008a). Accuracy of dementia diagnosis: a direct comparison between radiologists and a computerized method. *Brain*, 131(Pt 11):2969–2974.

Klöppel, S., Stonnington, C. M., Chu, C., Draganski, B., Scahill, R. I., Rohrer, J. D., Fox, N. C., Jack, Jr, C. R., Ashburner, J., and Frackowiak, R. S. J. (2008b). Automatic classification of MR scans in Alzheimer's disease. *Brain*, 131(Pt 3):681–689.

Lao, Z., Shen, D., Xue, Z., Karacali, B., Resnick, S. M., and Davatzikos, C. (2004). Morphological classification of brains via high-dimensional shape transformations and machine learning methods. *Neuroimage*, 21(1):46–57.

Last, D., Alsop, D. C., Abduljalil, A. M., Marquis, R. P., de Bazelaire, C., Hu, K., Cavallerano, J., and Novak, V. (2007). Global and regional effects of type 2 diabetes on brain tissue volumes and cerebral vasoreactivity. *Diabetes Care*, 30(5):1193–1199.

Laurén, J., Gimbel, D. A., Nygaard, H. B., Gilbert, J. W., and Strittmatter, S. M. (2009). Cellular prion protein mediates impairment of synaptic plasticity by amyloid-beta oligomers. *Nature*, 457(7233):1128–1132.

Lebel, C. and Beaulieu, C. (2011). Longitudinal development of human brain wiring continues from childhood into adulthood. *Journal of Neuroscience*, 31(30):10937–10947.

Lenroot, R. K. and Giedd, J. N. (2006). Brain development in children and adolescents: insights from anatomical magnetic resonance imaging. *Neuroscience and Biobehavioral Reviews*, 30(6):718–729.

Leow, A. D., Yanovsky, I., Parikshak, N., Hua, X., Lee, S., Toga, A. W., Jack, Jr, C. R., Bernstein, M. A., Britson, P. J., Gunter, J. L., Ward, C. P., Borowski, B., Shaw, L. M., Trojanowski, J. Q., Fleisher, A. S., Harvey, D., Kornak, J., Schuff, N., Alexander, G. E., Weiner, M. W., Thompson, P. M., and Alzheimer's Disease Neuroimaging Initiative (2009). Alzheimer's disease neuroimaging initiative: a one-year follow-up study using tensor-based morphometry correlating degenerative rates, biomarkers and cognition. *Neuroimage*, 45(3):645–655.

Liu, Y., Teverovskiy, L., Carmichael, O., Kikinis, R., Shenton, M., Carter, C., Stenger, V., Davis, S., Aizenstein, H., Becker, J., Lopez, O., and Meltzer, C. (2004). Discriminative MR image feature analysis for automatic schizophrenia and Alzheimer's disease classification. *Lecture Notes in Computer Science*, 3216:393–401.

Lu, P. H., Lee, G. J., Raven, E. P., Tingus, K., Khoo, T., Thompson, P. M., and Bartzokis, G. (2011). Age-related slowing in cognitive processing speed is associated with myelin integrity in a very healthy elderly sample. *Journal of Clinical and Experimental Neuropsychology*, 33(10):1059–1068.

Lu, P. H., Lee, G. J., Tishler, T. A., Meghpara, M., Thompson, P. M., and Bartzokis, G. (2013). Myelin breakdown mediates age-related slowing in cognitive processing speed in healthy elderly men. *Brain and Cognition*, 81(1):131–138.

Luchsinger, J. A. and Gustafson, D. R. (2009). Adiposity and Alzheimer's disease. *Current Opinion in Clinical Nutrition and Metabolic Care*, 12(1):15–21.

Luchsinger, J. A., Reitz, C., Honig, L. S., Tang, M. X., Shea, S., and Mayeux, R. (2005). Aggregation of vascular risk factors and risk of incident Alzheimer disease. *Neurology*, 65(4):545–551.

Mangialasche, F., Westman, E., Kivipelto, M., Muehlboeck, J.-S., Cecchetti, R., Baglioni, M., Tarducci, R., Gobbi, G., Floridi, P., Soininen, H., Kloszewska, I., Tsolaki, M., Vellas, B., Spenger, C., Lovestone, S., Wahlund, L.-O., Simmons, A., Mecocci, P., and AddNeuroMed consortium (2013). Classification and prediction of clinical diagnosis of Alzheimer's disease based on MRI and plasma measures of α-/γ-tocotrienols and γ-tocopherol. *Journal of Internal Medicine*, 273(6):602–621.

Marcus, D. S., Wang, T. H., Parker, J., Csernansky, J. G., Morris, J. C., and Buckner, R. L. (2007). Open Access Series of Imaging Studies (OASIS): cross-sectional MRI data in young, middle aged, nondemented, and demented older adults. *Journal of Cognitive Neuroscience*, 19(9):1498–1507.

Markus, H. S., Hunt, B., Palmer, K., Enzinger, C., Schmidt, H., and Schmidt, R. (2005). Markers of endothelial and hemostatic activation and progression of cerebral white matter hyperintensities: longitudinal results of the Austrian Stroke Prevention Study. *Stroke*, 36(7):1410–1414.

Marner, L., Nyengaard, J. R., Tang, Y., and Pakkenberg, B. (2003). Marked loss of myelinated nerve fibers in the human brain with age. *Journal of Comparative Neurology*, 462(2):144–152.

Martin, M., Schneider, R., Eicher, S., and Moor, C. (2012). The Functional Quality of Life (fQOL)-model. a new basis for quality of life-enhancing interventions in old age. *GeroPsych*, 25:33–40.

May, A. (2011). Experience-dependent structural plasticity in the adult human brain. *Trends in Cognitive Sciences*, 15(10):475–482.

McDonald, C. R., Gharapetian, L., McEvoy, L. K., Fennema-Notestine, C., Hagler, Jr, D. J., Holland, D., Dale, A. M., and Alzheimer's Disease Neuroimaging Initiative (2012). Relationship between regional atrophy rates and cognitive decline in mild cognitive impairment. *Neurobiology of Aging*, 33(2):242–253.

McLaughlin, K. A., Fox, N. A., Zeanah, C. H., Sheridan, M. A., Marshall, P., and Nelson, C. A. (2010). Delayed maturation in brain electrical activity partially explains the association between early environmental deprivation and symptoms of attention-deficit / hyperactivity disorder. *Biological Psychiatry*, 68(4):329–336.

Meda, S. A., Giuliani, N. R., Calhoun, V. D., Jagannathan, K., Schretlen, D. J., Pulver, A., Cascella, N., Keshavan, M., Kates, W., Buchanan, R., Sharma, T., and Pearlson, G. D. (2008). A large scale (n=400) investigation of gray matter differences in schizophrenia using optimized voxel-based morphometry. *Schizophrenia Research*, 101(1-3):95–105.

Meier-Ruge, W., Ulrich, J., Brühlmann, M., and Meier, E. (1992). Age-related white matter atrophy in the human brain. *Annals of the New York Academy of Sciences*, 673:260–269.

Middleton, L. E. and Yaffe, K. (2009). Promising strategies for the prevention of dementia. *Archives of Neurologyeurology*, 66(10):1210–1215.

Misra, C., Fan, Y., and Davatzikos, C. (2009). Baseline and longitudinal patterns of brain atrophy in MCI patients, and their use in prediction of short-term conversion to AD: results from ADNI. *Neuroimage*, 44(4):1415–1422.

Mohs, R. C. (1996). The Alzheimer's Disease Assessment Scale. *International Psychogeriatrics*, 8:195–203.

Mohs, R. C. and Cohen, L. (1988). Alzheimer's Disease Assessment Scale (ADAS). *Psychopharmacology Bulletin*, 24:627–628.

Moody, D. M., Thore, C. R., Anstrom, J. A., Challa, V. R., Langefeld, C. D., and Brown, W. R. (2004). Quantification of afferent vessels shows reduced brain vascular density in subjects with leukoaraiosis. *Radiology*, 233(3):883–890.

Morris, J. C. (1993). The Clinical Dementia Rating (CDR): current version and scoring rules. *Neurology*, 43(11):2412–2414.

Morrison, J. H. and Hof, P. R. (1997). Life and death of neurons in the aging brain. *Science*, 278(5337):412–419.

Mortel, K. F., Meyer, J. S., Herod, B., and Thornby, J. (1995). Education and occupation as risk factors for dementias of the Alzheimer and ischemic vascular types. *Dementia*, 6(1):55–62.

Muse, E. D., Jurevics, H., Toews, A. D., Matsushima, G. K., and Morell, P. (2001). Parameters related to lipid metabolism as markers of myelination in mouse brain. *Journal of Neurochemistry*, 76(1):77–86.

Neeb, H., Zilles, K., and Shah, N. J. (2006). Fully-automated detection of cerebral water content changes: study of age- and gender-related H2O patterns with quantitative MRI. *Neuroimage*, 29(3):910–922.

Nelson, P. T., Head, E., Schmitt, F. A., Davis, P. R., Neltner, J. H., Jicha, G. A., Abner, E. L., Smith, C. D., Van Eldik, L. J., Kryscio, R. J., and Scheff, S. W. (2011). Alzheimer's disease is not "brain aging": neuropathological, genetic, and epidemiological human studies. *Acta Neuropathology*, 121(5):571–587.

Nepal, B., Brown, L., and Ranmuthugala, G. (2010). Modelling the impact of modifying lifestyle risk factors on dementia prevalence in Australian population aged 45 years and over, 2006–2051. *Australasian Journal on Ageing*, 29(3):111–116.

Novak, V., Zhao, P., Manor, B., Sejdic, E., Alsop, D., Abduljalil, A., Roberson, P. K., Munshi, M., and Novak, P. (2011). Adhesion molecules, altered vasoreactivity, and brain atrophy in type 2 diabetes. *Diabetes Care*, 34(11):2438–2441.

Ohnishi, T., Matsuda, H., Tabira, T., Asada, T., and Uno, M. (2001). Changes in brain morphology in Alzheimer disease and normal aging: is Alzheimer disease an exaggerated aging process? *American Journal of Neuroradiology*, 22(9):1680–1685.

Oulhaj, A., Refsum, H., Beaumont, H., Williams, J., King, E., Jacoby, R., and Smith, A. D. (2010). Homocysteine as a predictor of cognitive decline in Alzheimer's disease. *International Journal of Geriatric Psychiatry*, 25(1):82–90.

Pakkenberg, B. and Gundersen, H. J. (1997). Neocortical neuron number in humans: effect of sex and age. *Journal of Comparative Neurology*, 384(2):312–320.

Pantoni, L., Garcia, J. H., and Gutierrez, J. A. (1996). Cerebral white matter is highly vulnerable to ischemia. *Stroke*, 27(9):1641–1647.

Paus, T., Keshavan, M., and Giedd, J. N. (2008). Why do many psychiatric disorders emerge during adolescence? *Nature Reviews Neuroscience*, 9(12):947–957.

Peskind, E. R., Li, G., Shofer, J., Quinn, J. F., Kaye, J. A., Clark, C. M., Farlow, M. R., DeCarli, C., Raskind, M. A., Schellenberg, G. D., Lee, V. M.-Y., and Galasko, D. R. (2006). Age and apolipoprotein E*4 allele effects on cerebrospinal fluid beta-amyloid 42 in adults with normal cognition. *Archives of Neurology*, 63(7):936–939.

Peters, R., Poulter, R., Warner, J., Beckett, N., Burch, L., and Bulpitt, C. (2008). Smoking, dementia and cognitive decline in the elderly, a systematic review. *BMC Geriatrics*, 8:36.

Pfefferbaum, A., Mathalon, D. H., Sullivan, E. V., Rawles, J. M., Zipursky, R. B., and Lim, K. O. (1994). A quantitative magnetic resonance imaging study of changes in brain morphology from infancy to late adulthood. *Archives of Neurology*, 51(9):874–887.

Pico, F., Dufouil, C., Lévy, C., Besancon, V., de Kersaint-Gilly, A., Bonithon-Kopp, C., Ducimetière, P., Tzourio, C., and Alpérovitch, A. (2002). Longitudinal study of carotid atherosclerosis and white matter hyperintensities: the EVA-MRI cohort. *Cerebrovascular Diseases*, 14(2):109–115.

Price, J. L., McKeel, Jr, D. W., Buckles, V. D., Roe, C. M., Xiong, C., Grundman, M., Hansen, L. A., Petersen, R. C., Parisi, J. E., Dickson, D. W., Smith, C. D., Davis, D. G., Schmitt, F. A., Markesbery, W. R., Kaye, J., Kurlan, R., Hulette, C., Kurland, B. F., Higdon, R., Kukull, W., and Morris, J. C. (2009). Neuropathology of nondemented aging: presumptive evidence for preclinical Alzheimer disease. *Neurobiology of Aging*, 30(7):1026–1036.

Price, J. L. and Morris, J. C. (1999). Tangles and plaques in nondemented aging and "preclinical" Alzheimer's disease. *Annals of Neurology*, 45(3):358–368.

Querbes, O., Aubry, F., Pariente, J., Lotterie, J.-A., Démonet, J.-F., Duret, V., Puel, M., Berry, I., Fort, J.-C., Celsis, P., and Alzheimer's Disease Neuroimaging Initiative (2009). Early diagnosis of Alzheimer's disease using cortical thickness: impact of cognitive reserve. *Brain*, 132(8):2036–2047.

Rajapakse, J. C., Giedd, J. N., and Rapoport, J. L. (1997). Statistical approach to segmentation of single-channel cerebral MR images. *IEEE Transactions on Medical Imaging*, 16(2):176–186.

Ramenghi, L. A., Martinelli, A., De Carli, A., Brusati, V., Mandia, L., Fumagalli, M., Triulzi, F., Mosca, F., and Cetin, I. (2011). Cerebral maturation in IUGR and appropriate for gestational age preterm babies. *Reproductive Sciences*, 18(5):469–475.

Raz, N. (2000). Aging of the brain and its impact on cognitive performance: Integration of structural and functional findings. In Craik, F. I. M. and Salthouse, T. A., editors, *Handbook of Aging and Cognition*, pages 1 – 90. Erlbaum, Mahwah, NJ.

Raz, N., Gunning-Dixon, F., Head, D., Rodrigue, K. M., Williamson, A., and Acker, J. D. (2004). Aging, sexual dimorphism, and hemispheric asymmetry of the cerebral cortex: replicability of regional differences in volume. *Neurobiology of Aging*, 25(3):377–396.

Raz, N., Gunning-Dixon, F. M., Head, D., Dupuis, J. H., and Acker, J. D. (1998). Neuroanatomical correlates of cognitive aging: evidence from structural magnetic resonance imaging. *Neuropsychology*, 12(1):95–114.

Raz, N., Lindenberger, U., Rodrigue, K. M., Kennedy, K. M., Head, D., Williamson, A., Dahle, C., Gerstorf, D., and Acker, J. D. (2005). Regional brain changes in aging healthy adults: general trends, individual differences and modifiers. *Cerebral Cortex*, 15(11):1676–1689.

Raz, N. and Rodrigue, K. M. (2006). Differential aging of the brain: patterns, cognitive correlates and modifiers. *Neuroscience and Biobehavioral Reviews*, 30(6):730–748.

Raz, N., Rodrigue, K. M., and Acker, J. D. (2003a). Hypertension and the brain: vulnerability of the prefrontal regions and executive functions. *Behavioral Neuroscience*, 117(6):1169–1180.

Raz, N., Rodrigue, K. M., Kennedy, K. M., Dahle, C., Head, D., and Acker, J. D. (2003b). Differential age-related changes in the regional metencephalic volumes in humans: a 5-year follow-up. *Neuroscience Letters*, 349(3):163–166.

Raz, N., Rodrigue, K. M., Kennedy, K. M., Head, D., Gunning-Dixon, F., and Acker, J. D. (2003c). Differential aging of the human striatum: longitudinal evidence. *American Journal of Neuroradiology*, 24(9):1849–1856.

Reijmer, Y. D., van den Berg, E., de Bresser, J., Kessels, R. P. C., Kappelle, L. J., Algra, A., Biessels, G. J., and Utrecht Diabetic Encephalopathy Study Group (2011). Accelerated cognitive decline in patients with type 2 diabetes: MRI correlates and risk factors. *Diabetes / Metabolism Research and Reviews*, 27(2):195–202.

Reisberg, B., Franssen, E. H., Hasan, S. M., Monteiro, I., Boksay, I., Souren, L. E., Kenowsky, S., Auer, S. R., Elahi, S., and Kluger, A. (1999). Retrogenesis: clinical, physiologic, and pathologic mechanisms in brain aging, Alzheimer's and other dementing processes. *European Archives of Psychiatry and Clinical Neuroscience*, 249 Suppl 3:28–36.

Resnick, S. M., Pham, D. L., Kraut, M. A., Zonderman, A. B., and Davatzikos, C. (2003). Longitudinal magnetic resonance imaging studies of older adults: a shrinking brain. *Journal of Neuroscience*, 23(8):3295–3301.

Richards, M. and Sacker, A. (2003). Lifetime antecedents of cognitive reserve. *Journal of Clinical and Experimental Neuropsychology*, 25(5):614–624.

Risacher, S. L., Saykin, A. J., West, J. D., Shen, L., Firpi, H. A., McDonald, B. C., and Alzheimer's Disease Neuroimaging Initiative (2009). Baseline MRI predictors of conversion from MCI to probable AD in the ADNI cohort. *Current Alzheimer Research*, 6(4):347–361.

Risacher, S. L., Shen, L., West, J. D., Kim, S., McDonald, B. C., Beckett, L. A., Harvey, D. J., Jack, Jr, C. R., Weiner, M. W., Saykin, A. J., and Alzheimer's Disease Neuroimaging Initiative (ADNI) (2010). Longitudinal MRI atrophy biomarkers: relationship to conversion in the ADNI cohort. *Neurobiology of Aging*, 31(8):1401–1418.

Rocchi, A., Pellegrini, S., Siciliano, G., and Murri, L. (2003). Causative and susceptibility genes for Alzheimer's disease: a review. *Brain Research Bulletin*, 61(1):1–24.

Rodrigue, K. M. and Raz, N. (2004). Shrinkage of the entorhinal cortex over five years predicts memory performance in healthy adults. *Journal of Neuroscience*, 24(4):956–963.

Saetre, P., Jazin, E., and Emilsson, L. (2011). Age-related changes in gene expression are accelerated in Alzheimer's disease. *Synapse*, 65(9):971–974.

Salat, D. H., Tuch, D. S., Greve, D. N., van der Kouwe, A. J. W., Hevelone, N. D., Zaleta, A. K., Rosen, B. R., Fischl, B., Corkin, S., Rosas, H. D., and Dale, A. M. (2005). Age-related alterations in white matter microstructure measured by diffusion tensor imaging. *Neurobiology of Aging*, 26(8):1215–1227.

Salerno, J. A., Murphy, D. G., Horwitz, B., DeCarli, C., Haxby, J. V., Rapoport, S. I., and Schapiro, M. B. (1992). Brain atrophy in hypertension. A volumetric magnetic resonance imaging study. *Hypertension*, 20(3):340–348.

Savva, G. M., Wharton, S. B., Ince, P. G., Forster, G., Matthews, F. E., and Brayne, C. (2009). Age, neuropathology, and dementia. *New England Journal of Medicine*, 360(22):2302–2309.

Scarmeas, N., Luchsinger, J. A., Schupf, N., Brickman, A. M., Cosentino, S., Tang, M. X., and Stern, Y. (2009). Physical activity, diet, and risk of Alzheimer disease. *JAMA*, 302(6):627–637.

Schmidt, R., Enzinger, C., Ropele, S., Schmidt, H., Fazekas, F., and Austrian Stroke Prevention Study (2003). Progression of cerebral white matter lesions: 6-year results of the Austrian Stroke Prevention Study. *Lancet*, 361(9374):2046–2048.

Schmidt, R., Launer, L. J., Nilsson, L.-G., Pajak, A., Sans, S., Berger, K., Breteler, M. M., de Ridder, M., Dufouil, C., Fuhrer, R., Giampaoli, S., Hofman, A., and CASCADE Consortium (2004). Magnetic resonance imaging of the brain in diabetes: the Cardiovascular Determinants of Dementia (CASCADE) study. *Diabetes*, 53(3):687–692.

Schölkopf, B. and Smola, A. (2002). *Learning with Kernels: Support Vector Machines, Regularization, Optimization, and Beyond*. MIT Press, Cambridge, Mass.

Schoonenboom, N. S. M., Reesink, F. E., Verwey, N. A., Kester, M. I., Teunissen, C. E., van de Ven, P. M., Pijnenburg, Y. A. L., Blankenstein, M. A., Rozemuller, A. J., Scheltens, P., and van der Flier, W. M. (2012). Cerebrospinal fluid markers for differential dementia diagnosis in a large memory clinic cohort. *Neurology*, 78(1):47–54.

Schwarz, C., Fletcher, E., DeCarli, C., and Carmichael, O. (2009). Fully-automated white matter hyperintensity detection with anatomical prior knowledge and without FLAIR. *Information Processing in Medical Imaging*, 21:239–251.

Selkoe, D. J. (2008). Soluble oligomers of the amyloid beta-protein impair synaptic plasticity and behavior. *Behavioural Brain Research*, 192(1):106–113.

Shankar, G. M., Li, S., Mehta, T. H., Garcia-Munoz, A., Shepardson, N. E., Smith, I., Brett, F. M., Farrell, M. A., Rowan, M. J., Lemere, C. A., Regan, C. M., Walsh, D. M., Sabatini, B. L., and Selkoe, D. J. (2008). Amyloid-beta protein dimers isolated directly from Alzheimer's brains impair synaptic plasticity and memory. *Nature Medicine*, 14(8):837–842.

Shaw, L. M., Vanderstichele, H., Knapik-Czajka, M., Clark, C. M., Aisen, P. S., Petersen, R. C., Blennow, K., Soares, H., Simon, A., Lewczuk, P., Dean, R., Siemers, E., Potter, W., Lee, V. M.-Y., Trojanowski, J. Q., and Alzheimer's Disease Neuroimaging Initiative (2009). Cerebrospinal fluid biomarker signature in Alzheimer's disease neuroimaging initiative subjects. *Annals of Neurology*, 65(4):403–413.

Shen, S., Sandoval, J., Swiss, V. A., Li, J., Dupree, J., Franklin, R. J. M., and Casaccia-Bonnefil, P. (2008). Age-dependent epigenetic control of differentiation inhibitors is critical for remyelination efficiency. *Nature Neuroscience*, 11(9):1024–1034.

Shields, S. A., Gilson, J. M., Blakemore, W. F., and Franklin, R. J. (1999). Remyelination occurs as extensively but more slowly in old rats compared to young rats following gliotoxin-induced CNS demyelination. *Glia*, 28(1):77–83.

Silk, T. J. and Wood, A. G. (2011). Lessons about neurodevelopment from anatomical magnetic resonance imaging. *Journal of Developmental and Behavioral Pediatrics*, 32(2):158–168.

Simic, G., Kostovic, I., Winblad, B., and Bogdanovic, N. (1997). Volume and number of neurons of the human hippocampal formation in normal aging and Alzheimer's disease. *Journal of Comparative Neurology*, 379(4):482–494.

Skullerud, K. (1985). Variations in the size of the human brain. influence of age, sex, body length, body mass index, alcoholism, Alzheimer changes, and cerebral atherosclerosis. *Acta Neurologica Scandinavica*, Supplement 102:1–94.

Sluimer, J. D., van der Flier, W. M., Karas, G. B., van Schijndel, R., Barnes, J., Boyes, R. G., Cover, K. S., Olabarriaga, S. D., Fox, N. C., Scheltens, P., Vrenken, H., and Barkhof, F. (2009). Accelerating regional atrophy rates in the progression from normal aging to Alzheimer's disease. *European Radiology*, 19(12):2826–2833.

Snowdon, D. A. (1997). Aging and Alzheimer's disease: lessons from the Nun Study. *Gerontologist*, 37(2):150–156.

Snowdon, D. A. (2003). Healthy aging and dementia: findings from the Nun Study. *Annals of Internal Medicine*, 139(5):450–454.

Solfrizzi, V., Capurso, C., D'Introno, A., Colacicco, A. M., Santamato, A., Ranieri, M., Fiore, P., Capurso, A., and Panza, F. (2008). Lifestyle-related factors in predementia and dementia syndromes. *Expert Review of Neurotherapeutics*, 8(1):133–158.

Solfrizzi, V., Scafato, E., Capurso, C., D'Introno, A., Colacicco, A. M., Frisardi, V., Vendemiale, G., Baldereschi, M., Crepaldi, G., Di Carlo, A., Galluzzo, L., Gandin, C., Inzitari, D., Maggi, S., Capurso, A., Panza, F., and Italian Longitudinal Study on Aging Working Group (2011). Metabolic syndrome, mild cognitive impairment, and progression to dementia. The Italian Longitudinal Study on Aging. *Neurobiology of Aging*, 32(11):1932–1941.

Spulber, G., Niskanen, E., MacDonald, S., Smilovici, O., Chen, K., Reiman, E. M., Jauhiainen, A. M., Hallikainen, M., Tervo, S., Wahlund, L.-O., Vanninen, R., Kivipelto, M., and Soininen, H. (2010). Whole brain atrophy rate predicts progression from MCI to Alzheimer's disease. *Neurobiology of Aging*, 31(9):1601–1605.

Steele, M., Stuchbury, G., and Münch, G. (2007). The molecular basis of the prevention of Alzheimer's disease through healthy nutrition. *Experimental Gerontology*, 42(1-2):28–36.

Stern, Y. (2002). What is cognitive reserve? Theory and research application of the reserve concept. *Journal of the International Neuropsychological Society*, 8(3):448–460.

Stern, Y. (2003). The concept of cognitive reserve: a catalyst for research. *Journal of Clinical and Experimental Neuropsychology*, 25(5):589–593.

Stern, Y. (2006). Cognitive reserve and Alzheimer disease. *Alzheimer Disease and Associated Disorders*, 20(3 Suppl 2):S69–574.

Stern, Y., Alexander, G. E., Prohovnik, I., Stricks, L., Link, B., Lennon, M. C., and Mayeux, R. (1995). Relationship between lifetime occupation and parietal flow: implications for a reserve against Alzheimer's disease pathology. *Neurology*, 45(1):55–60.

Stern, Y., Gurland, B., Tatemichi, T. K., Tang, M. X., Wilder, D., and Mayeux, R. (1994). Influence of education and occupation on the incidence of Alzheimer's disease. *JAMA*, 271(13):1004–1010.

Stern, Y., Habeck, C., Moeller, J., Scarmeas, N., Anderson, K. E., Hilton, H. J., Flynn, J., Sackeim, H., and van Heertum, R. (2005). Brain networks associated with cognitive reserve in healthy young and old adults. *Cerebral Cortex*, 15(4):394–402.

Stewart, R. and Liolitsa, D. (1999). Type 2 diabetes mellitus, cognitive impairment and dementia. *Diabetic Medicine*, 16(2):93–112.

Stonnington, C. M., Chu, C., Klöppel, S., Jack, Jr, C. R., Ashburner, J., Frackowiak, R. S. J., and Alzheimer Disease Neuroimaging Initiative (2010). Predicting clinical scores from magnetic resonance scans in Alzheimer's disease. *Neuroimage*, 51(4):1405–1413.

Strassburger, T. L., Lee, H. C., Daly, E. M., Szczepanik, J., Krasuski, J. S., Mentis, M. J., Salerno, J. A., DeCarli, C., Schapiro, M. B., and Alexander, G. E. (1997). Interactive effects of age and hypertension on volumes of brain structures. *Stroke*, 28(7):1410–1417.

Strozyk, D., Blennow, K., White, L. R., and Launer, L. J. (2003). CSF Abeta 42 levels correlate with amyloid-neuropathology in a population-based autopsy study. *Neurology*, 60(4):652–656.

Tan, Z. S., Beiser, A. S., Fox, C. S., Au, R., Himali, J. J., Debette, S., Decarli, C., Vasan, R. S., Wolf, P. A., and Seshadri, S. (2011). Association of metabolic dysregulation with volumetric brain magnetic resonance imaging and cognitive markers of subclinical brain aging in middle-aged adults: the Framingham Offspring Study. *Diabetes Care*, 34(8):1766–1770.

Teipel, S. J., Born, C., Ewers, M., Bokde, A. L. W., Reiser, M. F., Möller, H.-J., and Hampel, H. (2007). Multivariate deformation-based analysis of brain atrophy to predict Alzheimer's disease in mild cognitive impairment. *Neuroimage*, 38(1):13–24.

Terribilli, D., Schaufelberger, M. S., Duran, F. L. S., Zanetti, M. V., Curiati, P. K., Menezes, P. R., Scazufca, M., Amaro, Jr, E., Leite, C. C., and Busatto, G. F. (2011). Age-related gray matter volume changes in the brain during non-elderly adulthood. *Neurobiology of Aging*, 32(2):354–368.

Thompson, P. M., Hayashi, K. M., de Zubicaray, G., Janke, A. L., Rose, S. E., Semple, J., Herman, D., Hong, M. S., Dittmer, S. S., Doddrell, D. M., and Toga, A. W. (2003). Dynamics of gray matter loss in Alzheimer's disease. *Journal of Neuroscience*, 23(3):994–1005.

Thompson, P. M., Hayashi, K. M., Sowell, E. R., Gogtay, N., Giedd, J. N., Rapoport, J. L., de Zubicaray, G. I., Janke, A. L., Rose, S. E., Semple, J., Doddrell, D. M., Wang, Y., van Erp, T. G. M., Cannon, T. D., and Toga, A. W. (2004). Mapping cortical change in Alzheimer's disease, brain development, and schizophrenia. *Neuroimage*, 23 Suppl 1:S2–18.

Tipping, M. (2000). The relevance vector machine. In Solla, S., Leen, T., and Müller, K.-R., editors, *Advances in Neural Information Processing Systems.*, volume 12, pages 652–658. MIT Press.

Tipping, M. (2001). Sparse bayesian learning and the relevance vector machine. *Journal of Machine Learning Research*, 1:211–244.

Tipping, M. and Faul, A. (2003). Fast marginal likelihood maximisation for sparse bayesian models. In Bishop, C. and Frey, B., editors, *Proceedings of the Ninth International Workshop on Artificial Intelligence and Statistics*. Key West, FL.

Tobinick, E. L. and Gross, H. (2008). Rapid improvement in verbal fluency and aphasia following perispinal etanercept in Alzheimer's disease. *BMC Neurology*, 8:27.

Toga, A. W., Thompson, P. M., and Sowell, E. R. (2006). Mapping brain maturation. *Trends in Neurosciences*, 29(3):148–159.

Tohka, J., Zijdenbos, A., and Evans, A. (2004). Fast and robust parameter estimation for statistical partial volume models in brain MRI. *Neuroimage*, 23(1):84–97.

Tomlinson, D. R. and Gardiner, N. J. (2008). Glucose neurotoxicity. *Nature Reviews Neuroscience*, 9(1):36–45.

Trachtenberg, A. J., Filippini, N., Cheeseman, J., Duff, E. P., Neville, M. J., Ebmeier, K. P., Karpe, F., and Mackay, C. E. (2012). The effects of APOE on brain activity do not simply reflect the risk of Alzheimer's disease. *Neurobiology of Aging*, 33(3):618.e1–e13.

Tyas, S. L., Salazar, J. C., Snowdon, D. A., Desrosiers, M. F., Riley, K. P., Mendiondo, M. S., and Kryscio, R. J. (2007). Transitions to mild cognitive impairments, dementia, and death: findings from the Nun Study. *American Journal of Epidemiology*, 165(11):1231–1238.

Uylings, H. B. M. and de Brabander, J. M. (2002). Neuronal changes in normal human aging and Alzheimer's disease. *Brain and Cognition*, 49(3):268–276.

van der Maaten, L. (2007). An introduction to dimensionality reduction using MATLAB. Technical report MICC 07-07, Maastricht University, Maastricht, The Netherlands.

van der Maaten, L. (2008). MATLAB toolbox for dimensionality reduction.

Van Dijk, K. R. A., Sabuncu, M. R., and Buckner, R. L. (2012). The influence of head motion on intrinsic functional connectivity MRI. *Neuroimage*, 59(1):431–438.

van Elderen, S. G. C., de Roos, A., de Craen, A. J. M., Westendorp, R. G. J., Blauw, G. J., Jukema, J. W., Bollen, E. L. E. M., Middelkoop, H. A. M., van Buchem, M. A., and van der Grond, J. (2010). Progression of brain atrophy and cognitive decline in diabetes mellitus: a 3-year follow-up. *Neurology*, 75(11):997–1002.

Van Gerven, P. W. M., Van Boxtel, M. P. J., Ausems, E. E. B., Bekers, O., and Jolles, J. (2012). Do apolipoprotein E genotype and educational attainment predict the rate of cognitive decline in normal aging? A 12-year follow-up of the Maastricht Aging Study. *Neuropsychology*, 26(4):459–472.

van Swieten, J. C., Geyskes, G. G., Derix, M. M., Peeck, B. M., Ramos, L. M., van Latum, J. C., and van Gijn, J. (1991). Hypertension in the elderly is associated with white matter lesions and cognitive decline. *Annals of Neurology*, 30(6):825–830.

Velayudhan, L., Poppe, M., Archer, N., Proitsi, P., Brown, R. G., and Lovestone, S. (2010). Risk of developing dementia in people with diabetes and mild cognitive impairment. *British Journal of Psychiatry*, 196(1):36–40.

Vemuri, P., Gunter, J. L., Senjem, M. L., Whitwell, J. L., Kantarci, K., Knopman, D. S., Boeve, B. F., Petersen, R. C., and Jack, Jr, C. R. (2008). Alzheimer's disease diagnosis in individual subjects using structural MR images: validation studies. *Neuroimage*, 39(3):1186–1197.

Vemuri, P., Wiste, H. J., Weigand, S. D., Shaw, L. M., Trojanowski, J. Q., Weiner, M. W., Knopman, D. S., Petersen, R. C., Jack, Jr, C. R., and Alzheimer's Disease Neuroimaging Initiative (2009a). MRI and CSF biomarkers in normal, MCI, and AD subjects: diagnostic discrimination and cognitive correlations. *Neurology*, 73(4):287–293.

Vemuri, P., Wiste, H. J., Weigand, S. D., Shaw, L. M., Trojanowski, J. Q., Weiner, M. W., Knopman, D. S., Petersen, R. C., Jack, Jr, C. R., and Alzheimer's Disease Neuroimaging Initiative (2009b). MRI and CSF biomarkers in normal, MCI, and AD subjects: predicting future clinical change. *Neurology*, 73(4):294–301.

Verbruggen, K. T., Meiners, L. C., Sijens, P. E., Lunsing, R. J., van Spronsen, F. J., and Brouwer, O. F. (2009). Magnetic resonance imaging and proton magnetic resonance spectroscopy of the brain in the diagnostic evaluation of developmental delay. *European Journal of Paediatric Neurology*, 13(2):181–190.

Walhovd, K. B., Fjell, A. M., Brewer, J., McEvoy, L. K., Fennema-Notestine, C., Hagler, Jr, D. J., Jennings, R. G., Karow, D., Dale, A. M., and Alzheimer's Disease Neuroimaging Initiative (2010). Combining MR imaging, positron-emission tomography, and CSF biomarkers in the diagnosis and prognosis of Alzheimer disease. *AJNR*, 31(2):347–354.

Wang, P.-N., Liu, H.-C., Lirng, J.-F., Lin, K.-N., and Wu, Z.-A. (2009). Accelerated hippocampal atrophy rates in stable and progressive amnestic mild cognitive impairment. *Psychiatry Research*, 171(3):221–231.

Wang, Y., Fan, Y., Bhatt, P., and Davatzikos, C. (2010). High-dimensional pattern regression using machine learning: from medical images to continuous clinical variables. *Neuroimage*, 50(4):1519–1535.

Westman, E., Muehlboeck, J.-S., and Simmons, A. (2012). Combining MRI and CSF measures for classification of Alzheimer's disease and prediction of mild cognitive impairment conversion. *Neuroimage*, 62:229–238.

Westman, E., Simmons, A., Zhang, Y., Muehlboeck, J.-S., Tunnard, C., Liu, Y., Collins, L., Evans, A., Mecocci, P., Vellas, B., Tsolaki, M., Kloszewska, I., Soininen, H., Lovestone, S., Spenger, C., Wahlund, L.-O., and AddNeuroMed consortium (2011). Multivariate analysis of MRI data for

Alzheimer's disease, mild cognitive impairment and healthy controls. *Neuroimage*, 54(2):1178–1187.

Weston, J., Elisseeff, A., Bakir, G., and Sinz, F. (2006). *The Spider*. http://www.kyb.mpg.de/bs/people/spider/main.html.

Whalley, L. J., Staff, R. T., Murray, A. D., Duthie, S. J., Collins, A. R., Lemmon, H. A., Starr, J. M., and Deary, I. J. (2003). Plasma vitamin C, cholesterol and homocysteine are associated with grey matter volume determined by MRI in non-demented old people. *Neuroscience Letters*, 341(3):173–176.

Wilke, M. and Holland, S. K. (2003). Variability of gray and white matter during normal development: a voxel-based MRI analysis. *Neuroreport*, 14(15):1887–1890.

Williams, J. H., Pereira, E. A. C., Budge, M. M., and Bradley, K. M. (2002). Minimal hippocampal width relates to plasma homocysteine in community-dwelling older people. *Age and Ageing*, 31(6):440–444.

Wilson, R. S., Leurgans, S. E., Boyle, P. A., and Bennett, D. A. (2011). Cognitive decline in prodromal Alzheimer disease and mild cognitive impairment. *Archives of Neurology*, 68(3):351–356.

Wishart, H. A., Saykin, A. J., Rabin, L. A., Santulli, R. B., Flashman, L. A., Guerin, S. J., Mamourian, A. C., Belloni, D. R., Rhodes, C. H., and McAllister, T. W. (2006). Increased brain activation during working memory in cognitively intact adults with the APOE epsilon4 allele. *American Journal of Psychiatry*, 163(9):1603–1610.

Wolkowitz, O. M., Epel, E. S., Reus, V. I., and Mellon, S. H. (2010). Depression gets old fast: do stress and depression accelerate cell aging? *Depression and Anxiety*, 27(4):327–338.

Wolkowitz, O. M., Reus, V. I., and Mellon, S. H. (2011). Of sound mind and body: depression, disease, and accelerated aging. *Dialogues in Clinical Neuroscience*, 13(1):25–39.

Wolz, R., Julkunen, V., Koikkalainen, J., Niskanen, E., Zhang, D. P., Rueckert, D., Soininen, H., Lötjönen, J., and Alzheimer's Disease Neuroimaging Initiative (2011). Multi-method analysis of MRI images in early diagnostics of Alzheimer's disease. *PLoS One*, 6(10):e25446.

Woodruff-Pak, D. S., Vogel, R. W., Ewers, M., Coffey, J., Boyko, O. B., and Lemieux, S. K. (2001). MRI-assessed volume of cerebellum correlates with associative learning. *Neurobiology of Learning and Memory*, 76(3):342–357.

Xu, G., Liu, X., Yin, Q., Zhu, W., Zhang, R., and Fan, X. (2009). Alcohol consumption and transition of mild cognitive impairment to dementia. *Psychiatry and Clinical Neurosciences*, 63(1):43–49.

Xu, W. L., Qiu, C. X., Wahlin, A., Winblad, B., and Fratiglioni, L. (2004). Diabetes mellitus and risk of dementia in the Kungsholmen project: a 6-year follow-up study. *Neurology*, 63(7):1181–1186.

Yesavage, J. A. (1988). Geriatric Depression Scale. *Psychopharmacology Bulletin*, 24(4):709–711.

Zhan, W., Zhang, Y., Mueller, S. G., Lorenzen, P., Hadjidemetriou, S., Schuff, N., and Weiner, M. W. (2009). Characterization of white matter degeneration in elderly subjects by magnetic resonance diffusion and FLAIR imaging correlation. *Neuroimage*, 47 Suppl 2:T58–65.

Zhang, D., Wang, Y., Zhou, L., Yuan, H., Shen, D., and Alzheimer's Disease Neuroimaging Initiative (2011). Multimodal classification of Alzheimer's disease and mild cognitive impairment. *Neuroimage*, 55(3):856–867.

Zheng, Y.-T., Neo, S.-Y., Chua, T.-S., and Tian, Q. (2008). Probabilistic optimized ranking for multimedia semantic concept detection via RVM. In *Proceedings of the 2008 international conference on Content-based image and video retrieval. Niagara Falls, Canada*, 161–168. ACM.

Zimmet, P., Alberti, K. G., and Shaw, J. (2001). Global and societal implications of the diabetes epidemic. *Nature*, 414(6865):782–787.

Zylberstein, D. E., Lissner, L., Björkelund, C., Mehlig, K., Thelle, D. S., Gustafson, D., Ostling, S., Waern, M., Guo, X., and Skoog, I. (2011). Midlife homocysteine and late-life dementia in women. A prospective population study. *Neurobiology of Aging*, 32(3):380–386.

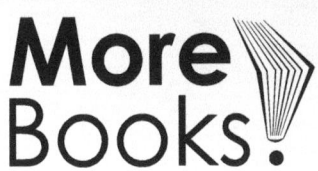

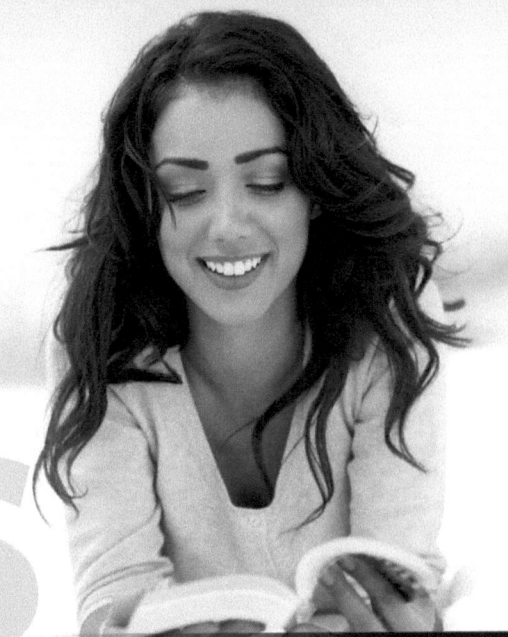

I want morebooks!

Buy your books fast and straightforward online - at one of the world's fastest growing online book stores! Environmentally sound due to Print-on-Demand technologies.

Buy your books online at
www.get-morebooks.com

Kaufen Sie Ihre Bücher schnell und unkompliziert online – auf einer der am schnellsten wachsenden Buchhandelsplattformen weltweit! Dank Print-On-Demand umwelt- und ressourcenschonend produziert.

Bücher schneller online kaufen
www.morebooks.de

VDM Verlagsservicegesellschaft mbH
Heinrich-Böcking-Str. 6-8
D - 66121 Saarbrücken

Telefax: +49 681 93 81 567-9

info@vdm-vsg.de
www.vdm-vsg.de

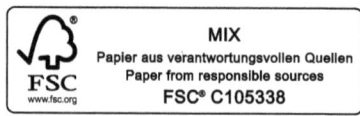

Printed by Books on Demand GmbH, Norderstedt / Germany